Gender Differences *in*

Gender differences
ar Disorders

From Bench to Bedside

Review of Psychiatry Series
John M. Oldham, M.D., and
Michelle B. Riba, M.D.
Series Editors

Gender Differences in Mood and Anxiety Disorders

From Bench to Bedside

EDITED BY

Ellen Leibenluft, M.D.

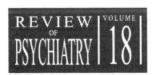

REVIEW OF PSYCHIATRY · VOLUME 18

No. 3

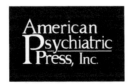

American Psychiatric Press, Inc.

Washington, DC
London, England

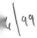

Copyright © 1999 American Psychiatric Press, Inc.

02 01 00 99   4 3 2 1

ALL RIGHTS RESERVED

Manufactured in the United States of America on acid-free paper

American Psychiatric Press, Inc.
1400 K Street, N.W.
Washington, DC   20005
www.appi.org

The correct citation for this book is

> Leibenluft E (ed.): *Gender Differences in Mood and Anxiety Disorders* (Review of Psychiatry Series; Oldham JO and Riba MB, series eds.). Washington, DC, American Psychiatric Press, 1999

Library of Congress Cataloging-in-Publication Data
Gender differences in mood and anxiety disorders : from bench to bedside / edited by Ellen Leibenluft.
     p.   cm. — (Review of psychiatry series ; v. 18, no. 3)
    Includes bibliographical references and index.
    ISBN 0-88048-958-8 (alk. paper)
    1. Affective disorders—Sex factors. 2. Anxiety—Sex factors. 3. Affective disorders—Endocrine aspects. 4. Anxiety—Endocrine aspects. 5. Affective disorders—Pathophysiology. 6. Anxiety—Pathophysiology.   I. Leibenluft, Ellen, 1953- . II. Series
    [DNLM: 1. Mood Disorders—pathophysiology. 2. Anxiety Disorders—pathophysiology. 3. Sex Hormones—physiology. 4. Sex Factors.   WM 171 G3248 1999]
  RC537.G455   1999
  616.85′27—dc21
  DNLM/DLC   99-10440
  for Library of Congress   CIP

British Library Cataloguing in Publication Data
A CIP record is available from the British Library.

Contents

Chapter 3

**Modulation of Anxiety by
Reproductive Hormones**   **53**
    Margaret Altemus, M.D., and
    Elizabeth Kagan Arleo, B.A.

Chapter 4

**Hormone Replacement and Oral
Contraceptive Therapy: Do They
Induce or Treat Mood Symptoms?**   **91**
    Kimberly A. Yonkers, M.D., and
    Karen D. Bradshaw, M.D.

Chapter 5
Modulation of Monoamine
Neurotransmitters by Estrogen:
Clinical Implications   **137**
Charles DeBattista, M.D., D.M.H.,
David Lawrence Smith, M.D., and
Alan F. Schatzberg, M.D.

Afterword   *161*
Ellen Leibenluft, M.D.

Index   *167*

Contributors

Margaret Altemus, M.D. Assistant Professor, Department of Psychiatry, Cornell University Medical College, New York, New York

Nancy C. Andreasen, M.D., Ph.D. Director, Mental Health Clinical Research Center, University of Iowa College of Medicine, Iowa City, Iowa

Elizabeth Kagan Arleo, B.A. Department of Psychiatry, Cornell University Medical College, New York, New York

Karen D. Bradshaw, M.D. Professor, Department of Obstetrics and Gynecology, The University of Texas Southwestern Medical Center, Dallas, Texas

Charles DeBattista, M.D., D.M.H. Assistant Professor, Department of Psychiatry and Behavioral Sciences, Stanford University School of Medicine, Stanford, California

Ania Korszun, M.D., Ph.D. Consultant Psychiatrist, Department of Psychological Medicine, University of Wales Medical School, Heath Park, Cardiff, United Kingdom

Ellen Leibenluft, M.D. Chief, Unit on Affective Disorders, Pediatric and Developmental Neuropsychiatry, National Institute of Mental Health, Bethesda, Maryland

Peg C. Nopoulos, M.D. Clinical Director, Mental Health Clinical Research Center, University of Iowa College of Medicine, Iowa City, Iowa

John M. Oldham, M.D. Director, New York State Psychiatric Institute; Dollard Professor and Vice Chairman, Department of Psychiatry, Columbia University College of Physicians and Surgeons, New York, New York

Michelle B. Riba, M.D.   Clinical Associate Professor of Psychiatry and Associate Chair for Education and Academic Affairs, Department of Psychiatry, University of Michigan Health System, Ann Arbor, Michigan

Alan F. Schatzberg, M.D.   Kenneth T. Norris Jr. Professor in Psychiatry and Behavioral Sciences; Chairman, Department of Psychiatry and Behavioral Sciences, Stanford University School of Medicine, Stanford, California

David Lawrence Smith, M.D.   NIMH Research Fellow, Department of Psychiatry and Behavioral Sciences, Stanford University School of Medicine, Stanford, California

Kimberly A. Yonkers, M.D.   Associate Professor, Department of Psychiatry, Yale University School of Medicine, New Haven, Connecticut

Elizabeth Young, M.D.   Professor, Department of Psychiatry, and Director of Mood Disorders Program, University of Michigan at Ann Arbor

Introduction to the Review of Psychiatry Series

John M. Oldham, M.D., and
Michelle B. Riba, M.D., Series Editors

As this century and millennium come to a close, it seems a universal impulse to pause and "take stock." Any time is a good time to do this, of course, but the big round number 2,000 just over the horizon seems a special one. It turns out to be, in our opinion, quite a good time for the field of psychiatry. Although a great deal more work lies ahead, we have made substantial progress in the fight for parity, with stronger partnerships having been built among clinicians, patients, families, and advocates. We are hopefully past the most extreme swing of the pendulum of managed care overcontrol, with a new, quite strong professional voice emerging to articulate and define evidence-based practice guidelines and best practices and to set performance standards and develop quality and outcome indicators for good clinical care.

The explosion of knowledge in neuroscience, meanwhile, only accelerates, with its accompanying breathtaking advances in technology. As more is learned about the circuitry of the brain, we obtain a clearer understanding of neurodevelopment gone awry in vulnerable populations such as those at risk to develop schizophrenia. But as we learn more about the brain's "hard-wiring," an entire frontier of information is unfolding, demonstrating an unprecedented plasticity of the brain. In turn, the sensitive, bidirectional interplay between biology and the environment becomes the name of the game.

In the context of these and many other features of our present landscape, we have chosen for this year's Annual Review a sampling of the latest knowledge and thinking from clinical practice and from the laboratory: 1) countertransference issues in psychiatric treatment, 2) disruptive behavior disorders in children and adolescents, 3) gender differences in mood and anxiety disorders,

4) masculinity and sexuality, and 5) molecular biology of schizophrenia.

We are grateful to our section editors and our authors, who worked hard and successfully to produce the text material. As well, we are indebted to Carol Nadelson, M.D., Claire Reinburg, Pamela Harley, Ron McMillen, and the entire American Psychiatric Press, Inc., staff. And the entire project would not have been possible without the steady help of Sam McGowan and Linda Gacioch.

Foreword

Ellen Leibenluft, M.D.

Gender differences in the prevalence of anxiety and mood disorders have been well documented. Epidemiological studies across a number of cultures consistently show that, beginning at puberty, major depression, dysthymia, and anxiety disorders are two to three times more common in women than in men (Kessler et al. 1994; Robins et al. 1984). In addition, both adolescent and adult females are more likely than age-matched males to develop posttraumatic stress disorder in response to a traumatic event (Breslau et al. 1998). Why these gender differences in risk exist is perhaps one of the more intriguing and important questions in clinical psychiatric research today: intriguing, because a deeper understanding of why women are more likely than men to experience anxiety and depression will inform us about the pathophysiology of these clinical syndromes; important, because such knowledge will improve our ability to design interventions that prevent and treat these illnesses.

While gender differences in the prevalence of mood and anxiety disorders are well established, the data with regard to gender differences in treatment response or course are both more limited and more controversial. In major depression, a number of studies have addressed the question of whether the presentation and course of the illness differ by gender. The literature is somewhat mixed, but most investigators do not find significant differences between depressed men and depressed women in their symptom profile, the likelihood that they will relapse, or the chronicity of their illness. For example, Zlotnick et al. (1996) found that depressed men and women had similar symptoms, social supports, life events, and course. Similarly, Simpson et al. (1997) found that depressed men and women did not differ either in their initial clinical presentation or in their course over the subsequent 15 years.

In contrast to this literature on major depression, there is rather consistent evidence that the symptomatology and course of anxiety disorders differ by gender. For example, men with panic disorder and agoraphobia are more likely than women with the same diagnosis to also meet criteria for alcoholism (Cox et al. 1993). And women with panic disorder and agoraphobia are more likely than men to relapse after achieving remission, a difference that remains significant even when the data are controlled for the higher rates of alcoholism among men (Yonkers et al. 1998).

In both major depression and anxiety disorders, the literature on gender differences in treatment response is surprisingly sparse. Evidence indicates that depressed women are less likely to respond to imipramine than paroxetine (Steiner et al. 1993). These data are consistent with earlier studies indicating that men are more likely than women to respond favorably to imipramine (reviewed in Yonkers et al. 1992). Unfortunately, there is virtually no literature addressing the question of whether men and women differ in their response to mood stabilizers and/or to antianxiety agents.

In addition to the clinical importance of these gender differences in the prevalence and course of mood and anxiety disorders, gender is also an important factor to consider in the psychiatric care of patients because of the known relationship between female reproductive milestones and psychiatric illnesses. For example, some women have mood cycles that vary systematically with the menstrual cycle (Rubinow and Roy-Byrne 1984), and some women with major depressive disorder experience exacerbations of their illness during certain phases of the menstrual cycle (Yonkers and White 1992). In addition, pregnancy and the postpartum period can affect the course of mood and anxiety disorders. For example, there is some evidence that panic disorder symptoms may lessen during pregnancy (Klein et al. 1995), whereas obsessive-compulsive disorder may be exacerbated during that time (Altshuler et al. 1998). Women with bipolar disorder are clearly at high risk of relapse during the postpartum period (Kendell et al. 1987), and there is evidence that the same may be true of women with a history of major depressive disorder

(Frank et al. 1987). Gonadal steroids are implicated in postpartum mood disorders by evidence indicating that these disorders may be treated effectively by estrogen (Gregoire et al. 1996). Finally, as detailed by Yonkers and Bradshaw in Chapter 4, there is evidence that the perimenopause may be associated with mood instability in a significant number of women and that exogenous hormones may be effective in relieving these mood symptoms.

The purpose of this book is to review current research that might ultimately explain these observed gender differences in disease prevalence, treatment response, and course and that might elucidate how female reproductive events affect the course of mood and anxiety disorders. The chapters draw on data from healthy control subjects and animal models as well as from clinical populations. Our purpose in reviewing both basic and clinical data is to inform our readers not only about where the field is, but also about where it is headed. Clinical psychiatric research is being revolutionized by insights derived from basic neuroscience (including but not limited to those related to genetic mechanisms) as well as by relatively new neuroimaging techniques. Increasingly sensitive techniques for structural neuroimaging, which allow us to study brain anatomy, are now being complemented by functional imaging techniques, including positron-emission tomography (PET) functional magnetic resonance imaging (fMRI), and magnetic resonance spectroscopy (MRS). These functional techniques make use of a variety of strategies to allow investigators to ascertain which brain structures become metabolically active when a subject performs a specific task. In this way, investigators can actually see the central nervous system at work; thus, the brain is no longer the "black box" that it had been until the relatively recent development of these techniques.

Reflecting the ever-increasing contribution of neuroimaging to psychiatric research, this volume begins with a review by Nopoulos and Andreasen of gender differences in brain structure and function (see Chapter 1, Gender Differences in Neuroimaging Findings). The question of whether there are structural, anatomic differences between men's and women's brains has been a subject of discussion and dissension since at least 1673, when Francois Poullain de la Barre, commenting on recent anatomic studies, stated that "the mind has no sex" (Schiebinger 1989). Not surprisingly, others argued to the contrary and generally prevailed. As Nopoulos and Andreasen note, earlier in this century the debate centered on whether the corpus callosum is larger in women than men and whether, if such a gender difference exists, it might form the structural basis for functional differences, with women possibly showing decreased brain laterality compared with men. Indeed, the fact that women are more likely than men to have preserved speech after strokes localized to the left temporoparietal region, as well as other data reviewed in the chapter, indicates that functional gender differences in brain laterality probably do exist. Data also indicate that boys and men probably have more cerebral volume than girls and women and that women may have higher cerebral blood flow than men, although the functional significance of these differences is currently unknown.

In their chapter, Nopoulos and Andreasen emphasize the plasticity of the brain, which responds both structurally and functionally to environmental influences and experiences. The latter can include an interpersonal interaction or the repeated experience of an affect such as sadness. Thus, psychological events can cause biological changes; nurture can physically alter nature. It therefore follows that, in trying to determine the pathogenesis of, for example, a depressive episode, the question is not whether the cause is "psychological" or "biological," but rather the relative and precise contributions of genetic and environmental factors (since both have biological sequelae) to the development of the illness.

With regard to environmental factors, stressful events are among those that are most relevant to the onset of clinical depression. Indeed, Kendler et al. (1995) have shown that women inherit not just depression per se, but also a propensity to respond to stressful events by becoming depressed. Specifically, these investigators found that a stressful event increased the risk of a subsequent depressive episode by 14% in women with a strong family history of depression but by only 6% in women without such a history. Data such as these, as well as the fact that hypercortisolemia is perhaps the best-documented biological finding in major depression, has precipitated a great deal of research on the role of the stress-responsive hypothalamic-pituitary-adrenal (HPA) axis in the pathophysiology of depression. In Chapter 2 (Women, Stress, and Depression: Sex Differences in Hypothalamic-Pituitary-Adrenal Axis Regulation), Young and Korszun review this literature and its relevance to the increased prevalence of major depression in women.

As Young and Korszun note, the abnormalities of the HPA axis that we have come to associate with major depression are more common in women than in men. That is, depressed women are more likely than depressed men to have elevated cortisol levels and to fail to suppress cortisol secretion in response to the administration of dexamethasone or other steroidal agents. Furthermore, both estrogen and progesterone appear to interfere with the normal feedback mechanisms of the HPA axis, meaning that the response to a stressful event may be more robust and long-lasting in females, both animal and human, than in males. Whether this gonadal steroid effect contributes to women's increased risk for depressive and anxiety disorders is a question worthy of further research.

Gonadal steroid effects on the HPA axis are only one of several mechanisms by which these hormones might influence the development and course of mood and anxiety disorders in women. Altemus and Arleo, in Chapter 3 (Modulation of Anxiety by Reproductive Hormones), discuss other routes by which estrogen, progesterone, oxytocin, and neurosteroids (i.e., steroids synthesized in the brain itself) may exert clinically relevant actions. (In extending their discussion beyond the usually considered gonadal steroids, estrogen and progesterone, to oxytocin, Altemus and Arleo remind us of the important fact that lactation may have clinically significant psychotropic effects in the mother [Altemus et al. 1995]). As each of these hormones receives more study, it becomes evident that the label "reproductive hormone" is really a misnomer, since the actions of these hormones are not limited to the regulation of reproductive function. In the case of estrogen and progesterone, receptors in the hypothalamus and preoptic area are primarily responsible for reproductive function and sexual behavior, but gonadal steroid receptors also exist in the limbic system, including the hippocampus, cingulate cortex, and particularly the amygdala. In addition, gonadal steroid receptors have been found in the basal ganglia, midbrain raphe (site of serotonin synthesis), locus coeruleus (site of noradrenergic synthesis), and basal forebrain (site of acetylcholine synthesis) (McEwen et al. 1997).

Of these extrahypothalamic estrogen receptors, those in the hippocampus have probably received the most study. Since the hippocampus is a major site for feedback regulation of the HPA axis, it is here that gonadal steroids may, as Young and Korszun describe in Chapter 2, inhibit cortisol's negative feedback on its own secretion. In addition, as Altemus and Arleo note in Chapter 3, estrogen receptors in the hippocampus have been shown to have effects on learning and memory that may be relevant not only to the pathogenesis (and prevention [Yaffe et al. 1998]) of dementing processes but also to the development of anxiety disorders in humans.

In considering the effects of gonadal steroids on the brain, it is important to remember that these effects vary according to the organism's developmental stage. A large body of animal literature indicates that estrogen administered in utero or perinatally has effects on brain structure that are not functionally evident until after the animal reaches puberty. These so-called organizational effects of gonadal steroids can be contrasted with their "activational" effects, which are short-term effects caused by circulating hormone postpubertally. Organizational effects are difficult to study in humans, since they can only be addressed in "experiments of nature" such as Turner's syndrome (Murphy et al. 1997) or congenital adrenal hyperplasia (Berenbaum and Resnick 1997) or in the results of such unfortunate occurrences as the exposure of human fetuses to diethylstilbestrol (DES) in utero (Pillard et al. 1993). It is therefore a challenge for clinical researchers to ascertain whether estrogen's organizational effects play a role in women's increased risk for major depression, which, as noted above, does not emerge until after puberty (Kessler et al. 1993). Recent data, reviewed by Altemus and Arleo, are intriguing in their suggestion that prenatal stress may have a more profound effect on the HPA axis in female than in male rats (McCormick et al. 1995).

Given the widespread distribution of gonadal steroid receptors in the brain, it is not surprising that the administration of exogenous estrogen or progesterone has complex effects on mood in women. This clinically important literature is reviewed in Chapter 4 (Hormone Replacement and Oral Contraceptive Therapy: Do They Induce or Treat Mood Symptoms?) by Yonkers and Bradshaw, who note that exogenous gonadal steroids have been presumed to both improve and worsen mood. Since these hormones are frequently prescribed to women in the peri- or postmenopausal period, it is important to distinguish the effects of fluctuating—and eventually diminishing—endogenous hormone levels from those of exogenous hormones. Yonkers and Bradshaw note that the literature generally supports the contention that whereas the menopause itself is not associated with a significant upsurge in the incidence of major depression, there is evidence that the perimenopause may be associated with an increase in relatively mild mood syndromes. And, while acknowledging the many inconsistencies in the literature, these authors conclude that the evidence overall supports the contention that exogenous estrogen does have mild mood-elevating effects in peri- and postmenopausal women. In addition, some data indicate that parenteral or transdermal estrogen preparations may be more effective in this regard than orally administered hormones. With regard to progesterone, the literature is quite limited and contradictory, but some studies indicate that progesterone may have mild adverse effects on mood.

Outside of perimenopause or menopause, exogenous gonadal steroids are usually prescribed to women in the form of oral contraception. Yonkers and Bradshaw note that the negative effects of oral contraceptives on mood have probably been somewhat overstated, so that even a retrospective history of late luteal dysphoric disorder is not a contraindication to the use of oral contraceptives. And, while the literature indicates significant interindividual variability in women's sensitivity to the psychotropic effects of exogenous gonadal steroids, overall the data indicate that hormones alone are unlikely to be an effective treatment for clinically significant depression at any stage of a woman's life.

Possible neurotransmitter effects that may explain estrogen's psychotropic effects have already been alluded to earlier in this Foreword, in noting that the principal sites of serotonin, norepinephrine, and acetylcholine synthesis are all brain regions where estrogen receptors have been found. The effects of estrogen on monoamine function, and the implications of these effects for pharmacotherapy, are reviewed in this volume's final chapter, by DeBattista, Smith, and Schatzberg (see Chapter 5, Modulation of Monoamine Neurotransmitters by Estrogen: Clinical Implications). They describe data indicating that estrogen modulates serotonergic function at many levels, with effects on synthesis, receptor number and binding, and synaptic reuptake. To add to the complexity of the situation, it also appears that serotonin's effects vary according to the brain region, dose, and time course studied. Although it is difficult to synthesize this complexity into one generalization, DeBattista and colleagues conclude that, overall, estrogen may have an augmenting effect on serotonin function. As they note, this conclusion is consistent with data indicating that premenopausal women may respond particularly well to serotonergically active medications and that estrogen supplementation may increase the efficacy of serotonergic antidepressants in menopausal women. However, this conclusion is contradictory to a PET study by Nishizawa et al. (1997), which showed that premenopausal women have significantly lower rates of serotonin synthesis than do men.

As DeBattista and colleagues note, the situation with dopamine is as complex as that with serotonin. That is, contradictory animal and in vitro data indicate that estrogen may either block or inhibit dopamine activity. However, it is estrogen's antidopaminergic effects that may be particularly relevant clinically, since schizophrenia appears to have a later onset and to take a more benign course in premenopausal women than in men. In addition, women appear to need lower doses of neuroleptic medication than do men, although there are a number of possible reasons for this disparity.

In conclusion, our intention in these chapters is to convey what we have learned, as well as what we have yet to learn, about the nature and causes of gender differences in mood and anxiety disorders. Research in this area has increased markedly in recent years, so that many neglected research questions are now receiving considerable attention from both basic and clinical researchers. This is as it should be, because research into gender- and sex-related questions provides a window into both normal brain function and pathophysiology and can ultimately improve our ability to treat patients who suffer from these serious illnesses.

References

Altemus M, Deuster P, Galliven E, et al: Suppression of hypothalamic-pituitary-adrenal axis responses to stress in lactating women. J Clin Endocrinol Metab 80:2954–2959, 1995

Altshuler L, Hendrick V, Cohen L: Course of mood and anxiety disorders during pregnancy and the postpartum period. J Clin Psychiatry 59:29–33, 1998

Berenbaum SA, Resnick SM: Early androgen effects on aggression in children and adults with congenital adrenal hyperplasia. Psychoneuroendocrinology 22:505–515, 1997

Breslau N, Kessler RC, Chilcoat HD, et al: Trauma and posttraumatic stress disorder in the community: the 1996 Detroit area survey of trauma. Arch Gen Psychiatry 55:626–632, 1998

Cox BJ, Swinson RP, Shulman ID, et al: Gender effects and alcohol use in panic disorder with agoraphobia. Behav Res Ther 31:413–416, 1993

Frank E, Kupfer D, Jacob M, et al: Pregnancy-related affective episodes among women with recurrent depression. Am J Psychiatry 144:288–293, 1987

Gregoire AJ, Kumar R, Everitt B, et al: Transdermal oestrogen for treatment of severe postnatal depression. Lancet 347:930–933, 1996

Kendell RE, Chalmers JC, Platz C: Epidemiology of puerperal psychoses. Br J Psychiatry 150:662–673, 1987

Kendler KS, Kessler RC, Walters EE, et al: Stressful life events, genetic liability, and onset of an episode of depression in women. Am J Psychiatry 152:833–842, 1995

Kessler R, McGonagle K, Swartz M, et al: Sex and depression in the National Comorbidity Survey, I: lifetime prevalence, chronicity, and recurrence. J Affect Disord 29:85–96, 1993

Kessler RC, McGonagle KA, Zhao S, et al: Lifetime and 12-month prevalence of DSM-III-R psychiatric disorders in the United States. Arch Gen Psychiatry 51:8–19, 1994

Klein D, Skrobala A, Garfinkel R: Preliminary look at the effects of pregnancy on the course of panic disorder. Anxiety 1:227–232, 1995

McCormick C, Smythe J, Sharma S, et al: Sex-specific effects of prenatal stress on hypothalamic-pituitary-adrenal responses to stress and brain glucocorticoid receptor density in adult rats. Brain Res Dev Brain Res 84:55–61, 1995

McEwen BS, Alves SE, Bulloch K, et al: Ovarian steroids and the brain: implications for cognition and aging. Neurology 48 (suppl 7):S8–S15, 1997

Murphy DGM, Mentis MJ, Pietrini P, et al: A PET study of Turner's syndrome: effects of sex steroids and the X chromosome on the brain. Biol Psychiatry 41:285–298, 1997

Nishizawa S, Benkelfat C, Young SN, et al: Differences between males and females in rates of serotonin synthesis in human brain. Proc Natl Acad Sci U S A 94:5308–5313, 1997

Pillard RC, Rosen LR, Meyer-Bahlburg H, et al: Psychopathology and social functioning in men prenatally exposed to diethylstilbestrol (DES). Psychosom Med 55:485–491, 1993

Robins L, Helzer J, Weissman M, et al: Lifetime prevalence of specific psychiatric disorders in three sites. Arch Gen Psychiatry 41:949–958, 1984

Rubinow D, Roy-Byrne P: Premenstrual syndromes: overviews from a methodologic perspective. Am J Psychiatry 141:163–172, 1984

Schiebinger L: The Mind Has No Sex: Women in the Origins of Modern Science. Cambridge, MA, Harvard University Press, 1989

Simpson H, Nee J, Endicott J: First-episode major depression: few sex differences in course. Arch Gen Psychiatry 54:633–639, 1997

Steiner M, Wheadon DE, Krieder MS, et al: Antidepressant response to paroxetine by gender. Paper presented at the 146th Annual Meeting of the American Psychiatric Association, San Francisco, CA, May 1993

Yaffe K, Sawaya G, Lieberburg I, et al: Estrogen therapy in postmenopausal women: effects on cognitive function and dementia. JAMA 279:688–695, 1998

Yonkers KA, White K: Premenstrual exacerbation of depression: one process or two? J Clin Psychiatry 53:289–292, 1992

Yonkers KA, Kando JC, Cole JO, et al: Gender differences in pharmacokinetics and pharmacodynamics of psychotropic medication. Am J Psychiatry 149:587–595, 1992

Yonkers KA, Zlotnick C, Allsworth J, et al: Is the course of panic disorder the same in women and men? Am J Psychiatry 155:596–602, 1998

Zlotnick C, Shea M, Pilkonis P, et al: Gender, type of treatment, dysfunctional attitudes, social support, life events, and depressive symptoms over naturalistic follow-up. Am J Psychiatry 153:1021–1027, 1996

Chapter 1

Gender Differences in Neuroimaging Findings

Peg C. Nopoulos, M.D., and
Nancy C. Andreasen, M.D., Ph.D.

In recent years, interest in the effects of gender on brain morphology has increased concomitantly with the rapid evolution of technology for brain imaging. The reasons for the increased interest are multiple. First is the search for a more thorough understanding of how brain structure and function differ (if at all) between the sexes. Second, an understanding of how brain morphology differs between the sexes is crucial in informing scientists how to control for sex effects when studying brain structure and function affected by disease processes. For example, when studying morphological brain changes resulting from a specific illness, such as schizophrenia, researchers must account for the differences between male and female brains; otherwise, these sex effects may potentially "wash out" any effect of disease pathology. A third reason for the increased interest in the effects of gender on brain morphology is the need to better understand how sex differences in the brain interact with disease pathology to produce the between-sex differences in disease phenomenology (e.g., presentation, course, severity, treatment response) that are observed in most neuropsychiatric disorders.

Despite the huge advances in the neurosciences over the last 10–20 years, the sum total of all the knowledge accumulated to date does not compare with what we do not yet know about the brain. The search for a better understanding of the human brain is a daunting task in and of itself, even without trying to sort out the effects of gender. Furthermore, identifying differences between the brains of men and women can have unintended consequences. Although such differences are intriguing, "difference" is often construed as a dichotomy of superiority versus inferiority.

An additional difficulty in the study of sex differences in the human brain is how to account for environmental influences. The brain is quite "plastic" and responds both structurally and functionally to environmental influences. From the time of birth, assigned gender imparts different treatment and expectations from parents, society, and culture. However, studies of neonates show sex differences in a variety of measures, including sensory responsiveness (Korner 1973), motor strength (Jacklin et al. 1981), pattern (Feldman et al. 1980) and symmetry of motor movement (Grattan et al. 1992), vocalization, visual acuity (Restak 1979), and eye contact time (Hittelman and Dickes 1979). These studies in neonates minimize if not eliminate social and environmental confounders and suggest the existence of a substrate of biological sex differences in brain–behavior relationships.

The second reason for the increased interest in sex differences in the brain—to better inform scientists how to control for sex differences when studying the effects of disease pathology—is critical to the study of any illness involving the brain. In the research of brain-based diseases, the prime objective is to understand how a particular disease manifests in brain structure and function so as to identify a specific pathoetiology. Yet in most neuropsychiatric illnesses the changes in brain morphology are actually quite subtle, and any sex effects that may exist could potentially mask the effect of the illness on the brain. For instance, our group and others have reported that patients with schizophrenia have smaller cerebral volumes than do healthy control subjects (Andreasen et al. 1994). The difference between groups is rather small (3.7%), however. In contrast, the difference in overall cerebral volume between the sexes has consistently been documented to be around 9%–10%. The magnitude of this difference highlights the importance of controlling for the effects of sex when examining brain morphology for disease effects. The large confound of sex can very easily "wash out" any effect of pathology.

For whatever reason, the tools provided by improved technology in structural and functional imaging have renewed interest in exploring sex differences in the brain. *Structural imaging* refers to methods that examine the structure or morphology of the human brain with either computed tomography (CT) or magnetic resonance imaging (MRI). *Functional imaging* refers to methods used to evaluate either blood flow or metabolism in the brain—measures interpreted as indicating specific brain activity. Functional imaging methods include single photon emission computed tomography (SPECT), positron-emission tomography (PET), and functional magnetic resonance imaging (fMRI). In this chapter we attempt to review and summarize the relevant findings of published brain-imaging studies of sex differences. As will be seen, the literature is young and therefore relatively scant. Unfortunately, there are many conflicting reports, and, as often occurs, the literature may be prone to bias from unpublished negative studies.

Researchers who study the brain have become increasingly aware of how important it is to employ a developmental perspective—that is, from gestation through old age. Therefore, this chapter is organized to review sex differences in brain structure and function from a life-cycle perspective.

Early Brain Development

Although a large amount of work has been done on the neurodevelopment of nonhuman mammals, many unanswered questions remain. Very little is known about the details of human brain development, including gender differences in the developmental process. One area of intensive research has been the effects of sex hormones on the developing brain. Most of the studies in this area have been conducted in rats and other nonhuman mammals. Although animal models provide framework and theory, our knowledge of the developmental effects of sex hormones in the human brain is still quite preliminary.

Effect of Sex Hormones on the Developing Fetus

Until about 6 weeks of gestation, male and female embryos have undifferentiated gonads and are morphologically identical. If there is a Y chromosome present, testes develop. If no Y chromosome is present, ovaries develop. Between 9 and 18 weeks, androgens secreted by fetal testes differentiate the fetus as male. Thus, once the sex of the gonads is determined, sexual differentiation of the rest of the body proceeds. Furthermore, this differentiation is directly influenced by the hormones secreted from the gonads and therefore is only indirectly related to genetic makeup. For example, the genotype of an embryo that is male would develop testes. However, if the testes do not produce testosterone, or if the testosterone is in some way ineffective on the tissues, the fetus develops as a phenotypic female, regardless of male genetic makeup. Conversely, if a genetically female fetus is exposed to testosterone at the right time in development, a phenotypic male will result.

Thus, it is the influence of sex hormones on undifferentiated fetal tissues during a "critical period" that results in sexual differentiation of the human *body*. This then invites the following question: Does the influence of sex hormones on the developing fetus result in sexual differentiation of the *brain?*

Effect of Sex Hormones on the Developing Brain

Studies in Nonhuman Mammals

For nonhuman mammals, the answer to the above question is yes. There exists an extensive body of published studies in nonhuman samples showing that the hormones present at a critical stage in brain development result in sexual dimorphism in both structure and function of the brain. With regard to brain structure, sex differences have been demonstrated at all structural levels including 1) gross volume of brain areas, 2) morphology of individual neurons, and 3) type and number of synapses (MacLusky and Naftolin 1981; Pilgrim and Hutchinson 1994). The effects of early exposure to sex hormones are considered to be "organizational" because they appear to alter brain function in a permanent fashion and are mediated by testosterone. Though most of the differences have been reported in the hypothalamus, the area of the brain governing sexual drive and behavior, differences have also been found in the amygdala and the cerebral cortex (Kawata 1995).

Studies in Humans

The evidence supporting the effect of early sex hormones on the human brain is much less direct. The critical developmental period for the fetal brain in humans is estimated to occur in early or midgestation, a time closely corresponding to the period when hormonal effects induce gonadal differentiation (Reinisch et al. 1979). Androgen levels in the male fetus remain high for at least 2 weeks after development of the genitalia, suggesting that this may be the period for "sexual differentiation of the brain." Studies showing that the fetal hypothalamus takes up radioactivity from labeled testosterone between 14 and 18 weeks support this hypothesis (Abramovich and Rowe 1973).

Due to obvious ethical concerns, scientists are unable to directly manipulate hormones early in gestation in humans. However, there are cases whereby "experiments of nature" allow indirect study of the effects of sex hormones on the developing brain and subsequent behavior. The effects of androgens (or lack thereof) on the developing brain were examined in a group of subjects with testicular feminization syndrome. These subjects are genetically male but phenotypically female (and thus raised as girls) because they are insensitive to the effects of androgen. One study found the subjects' cognitive pattern to be "typically female," with strengths in language and relative weaknesses in spatial orientation (Masica et al. 1969). This suggests that the lack of androgens allowed the brain to "differentiate" into a female one with typical female cognitive patterns. Conversely, females who have been exposed in utero to virilizing sex hormones (e.g., in congenital adrenal hyperplasia, or because of the mother's ingestion of diethylstilbestrol) have been shown to have superior visual-spatial abilities (a cognitive ability in which men typically outperform women) (Resnick et al. 1986) and increased left-hand preference (Geschwind and Galaburda 1985); in addition, they are more likely to be homosexual or bisexual than nonexposed females (Ehrhardt et al. 1985). Although these studies suggest that exposure to sex hormones shapes behaviors later in life, there is still very little evidence in the study of humans to make any definitive conclusions on this topic.

Brain Growth and Maturation

It has been suggested that human brain growth and maturation is a process that continues many years past birth, into adolescence and even adulthood. To understand the volumetric changes seen in the developing brain, a brief review of the development of the cellular structure of the brain may be helpful.

The development of the neuronal elements of the neocortex advances through a "progressive" mode, which is succeeded by a "regressive" mode of development. Neuronal division and migration is completed between 24 and 32 weeks of gestation in human cortex (Carlson et al. 1988). Neurons stop dividing when migration occurs. However, more than half of these neurons normally die after migration by a regressive process that appears to involve competition for trophic factors or interactions with a variety of types of targets (as opposed to programmed cell death) (Hamburger 1980). Most neuronal cell death occurs prenatally. An additional regressive developmental process is that of axon collateral and synapse elimination, often referred to as *pruning* (Purves and Lichtman 1985). In contrast to neuronal elimination, which occurs prenatally, this process starts prenatally but continues into childhood and adolescence, and is therefore considered a "late developmental" event. With regard to white matter, there appears to be only a progressive process by which enlargement and proliferation of glial elements form myelin. This process, however, is also quite prolonged, with some regions continuing to mature/myelinate through the third decade of life (Benes et al. 1994).

These histological changes have been corroborated by neuroimaging studies of brain development using MRI. An MRI study by Jernigan and Tallal (1990) confirmed that the volume of cortical gray matter declines through late childhood, as does the ratio of gray matter to white matter. Moreover, the reduction of the proportion of the cortical gray matter was found to be associated with an increase in ventricular cerebrospinal fluid.

Although neuroimaging techniques such as MRI have been available for many years, it is only recently that neuroimaging has been used to study the development of the normal human brain. MRI studies evaluating morphological brain changes throughout development report interesting sexual dimorphisms. Caviness et al. (1996) examined the brains of 15 males and 15 females ages 7–11 years, comparing them with the brains of a sample of 20 (10 male, 10 female) young adults. They found that the brain of the female child was 93% of the volume of the brain of the male child and that approximately 70% of this difference was attributable to the greater volume of central white matter in the male cerebrum, with the remainder of the difference attributable to a larger cerebellar volume in the male. These findings were in contrast to those of Reiss et al. (1996), who studied 85 healthy children ages 5–17 years. Although Reiss and colleagues found similar increases in total cerebral volume in boys compared with girls (10%), they found that increased cortical gray matter was the primary contributor to the larger brain volume in boys.

In the Caviness et al. (1996) study, the difference in brain tissue volume between girls and boys seemed to be generalized for the major regions of the brain (e.g., the lobes). Exceptions to this pattern were that in the female brains, the caudate, hippocampus, and pallidum were disproportionately large, whereas the amygdala was disproportionately small. These findings were similar to those of Giedd et al. (1996), who used MRI to study a total of 104 healthy children ages 4–18 years. The males had cerebral volumes that were 9% larger than those of the females, and as in the study by Caviness et al. (1996), this was a generalized effect with regard to the cerebral subdivisions. Also like Caviness et al., Giedd and colleagues found that the caudate volume in the female brain was disproportionately large, although, in contrast to the results of the Caviness et al. study, Giedd et al. found the globus pallidus and putamen to be proportionately larger in the male brain.

In addition to these cross-sectional differences in morphology between the sexes, the effects of age and maturational processes were examined in both the Caviness et al. (1996) and the Giedd et al. (1996) studies. The findings were complementary. Caviness et al. (1996) reported that in girls, the collective subcortical gray-matter structures of the forebrain are already at their adult volumes, whereas in boys, the volumes of these structures are greater than their adult volumes and thus, by implication, must "regress" in volume before adulthood. The study by Giedd et al. (1996) supported this assumption by reporting that caudate and putamen volumes decreased over time (between ages 4 and 18 years) in males but not in females. In addition, they showed that ventricular volume increased with age, especially after age 11 years, but, once again, only for the males. This increase in ventricle volume could be postulated as an *ex vacuo* process related to the decreased volume of the basal ganglia structures that lie in such close proximity to the lateral ventricles.

As stated by Caviness et al. (1996), "these juxtaposed progressive and regressive patterns of growth of brain structures implied by these observations in the human brain have a soundly established precedent in the developing rhesus brain" (p. 726). These changes in the brain, which are considered to be late developmental processes, are not subtle and can change the morphology of the brain significantly; for this reason, it is important to understand them better. Furthermore, these processes may be key to the pathoetiology of some neuropsychiatric illnesses. For example, several authors have considered the late-developmental regressive process of pruning in the cerebral cortex to be important in the pathology of schizophrenia (Feinberg 1982; Keshavan et al. 1994).

The Adult Brain

Sex Differences in Structural Morphology

Both autopsy (Dekaban and Sadowski 1978; Ho et al. 1980) and neuroimaging studies (Filipek et al. 1994; Pfefferbaum et al. 1994) have consistently documented differences in overall brain volume between the sexes, with the male brain being approximately 10% larger than the female brain. Although some of the authors of earlier studies argued that the larger brain volume in males than in females is due to sex differences in body size, the consensus in the literature at present is that this effect is independent of the difference in body size between the sexes. As discussed earlier in this chapter, this gender difference in brain size is also apparent in the developing brain, as shown by imaging studies in children and adolescents that report the male brain to be anywhere from 7% to 10% larger than the female brain (Caviness et al. 1996; Giedd et al. 1996; Reiss et al. 1996).

However, whether the increased size is related to a generalized or regional increase in volume has not been fully investigated. In a recent study from our center, MRI was used to evaluate brain morphology in 42 healthy females matched with 42 healthy males by age and IQ (P. C. Nopoulos, M. Flaum, and N. C. Andreasen, "Gender Differences in Brain Morphology: Regional Measures, Tissue Composition, and Surface Anatomy," April 1999 [unpublished study]). Using an automated imaging processing procedure, we obtained volumes for frontal lobe, parietal lobe, occipital lobe, temporal lobe, subcortical tissue, and cerebellum from a stereotaxic atlas (Talairach and Tournoux 1988; see Figure 1–1). Table 1–1 shows the results of the analysis of covariance (ANCOVA) used to evaluate the differences in global and regional brain volumes between the sexes. To control for differences in body size between the sexes, height was used as a covariate. Several measures, including cerebral tissue volume, showed a significant sex-by-height interaction, indicating that the relationship between height and cerebral tissue volume differed between the sexes (see subsection below titled "Sex Differences in the Relationship Between Brain Growth and Body Growth"). When significant, this interaction term was also accounted for in the analysis (see Table 1–1). A significant sex effect was found for cerebral tissue volume as a whole as well as for the volumes of each of the cerebrum's four lobes (frontal, temporal, parietal, and occipital). For all of these measures, males had larger volumes than females. Moreover, males' enlargement of cerebral tissue was generalized and did not appear to affect the volume of any one particular lobe. This confirms the findings of other studies in both adults (Murphy et al. 1996) and children (Giedd et al. 1996) that found no significant regional differences between male and female cerebral lobe volumes.

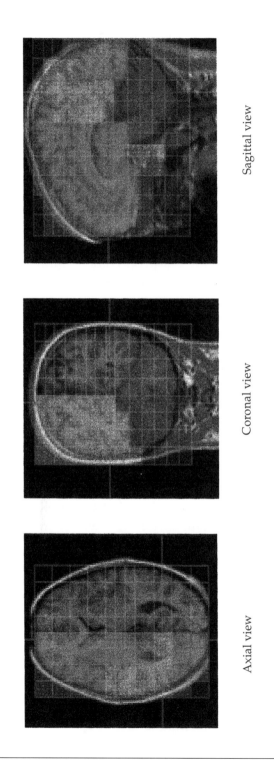

Figure 1–1. Talairach and Tournoux (1988) stereotaxic atlas–based method for automated measures of brain tissue volume. *Legend:* Blue = frontal lobe; white = temporal lobe; yellow = parietal lobe; green = occipital lobe; purple = cerebellum; red = subcortical tissue.

Sagittal view

Coronal view

Axial view

Table 1-1. Comparison of general and regional brain tissue volumes between the sexes

	Males ($n = 42$)		Females ($n = 42$)		Sex effect	
	Mean (SD)	Adjusted mean	Mean (SD)	Adjusted mean	F*	P
Cerebral tissue	1490.4 (116.7)	1256.8	1351.5 (112.80)	1167.1	3.84	.05
Subcortical tissue	58.0 (6.2)	57.8	53.9 (6.7)	55.1	1.37	.24
Cerebellar tissue	148.9 (19.6)	141.8	139.3 (14.4)	145.2	0.42	.51
Frontal lobe	459.9 (43.9)	458.6	409.8 (43.7)	426.7	4.49	.03
Temporal lobe	238.3 (19.9)	235.0	216.9 (19.2)	222.3	4.00	.04
Parietal lobe	268.9 (23.1)	271.9	242.6 (19.9)	249.0	4.21	.04
Occipital lobe	136.6 (18.6)	129.3	122.1 (15.4)	129.4	4.46	.03

Note. F = F distribution. * Analysis of covariance (ANCOVA) using height as covariate.

Although the sex differences in cerebral tissue volume remained after height was controlled, no significant differences were found in the volume of subcortical tissue, an area that includes the basal ganglia structures and other deep nuclei such as the thalamus. Given that males have larger cerebral volumes than females, this failure to find a sex effect on subcortical tissue volume is in accord with the results of other studies that have found subcortical structures such as the caudate nucleus to be proportionately larger in the brains of female adults (Filipek et al. 1994; Murphy et al. 1996) and of female children/adolescents (Caviness et al. 1996; Giedd et al. 1996; Reiss et al. 1996) than in the male brain. Murphy et al. (1996) also found the thalamus to be proportionately larger in the female brain.

Cerebellar tissue volume was also found not to differ between the sexes after controlling for height. This was a curious finding and somewhat unexpected. One possible interpretation is that the cerebellum does not vary in volume as much as the cerebrum does. The cerebellum is an interesting structure that accounts for only 10% of the average total brain weight (Blinkow and Glezer 1968) yet contains more than half of all neurons in the brain (Ghez 1991). Thus, it is a very compact structure that may not vary much in its overall volume.

Sex Differences in Tissue Composition

Sex effects on the relative composition of brain tissue—that is, the ratio of gray matter, white matter, and cerebrospinal fluid to total volume—have not been studied very thoroughly. Two recent MRI studies of adult brains supported the finding of Caviness et al. (1996) that in children's brains the volume differences between the sexes were at least partially accounted for by a relative increase in white matter in boys' brains (Filipek et al. 1994; Passe et al. 1997). Also, an MRI study by Schlaepfer et al. (1995) found that the percentages of gray matter in the dorsolateral prefrontal cortex and the superior temporal gyrus in women were 23.2% and 12.8% greater, respectively, than those in men. These increases in gray matter in the female brain were found in cortical areas related to language, suggesting a biological correlate of the behavioral finding that women perform better than men on verbal-ability tasks. Schlaepfer and colleagues also postulated that the regional increases in percentage of gray matter among females may account for findings of higher cerebral blood flow in women compared with men reported by several groups (for a review, see R. E. Gur and R. C. Gur 1990) by virtue of the fact that gray matter is more highly vascularized than white matter.

Sex Differences in the Relationship Between Brain Growth and Body Growth

An unexpected and interesting finding from a neuroimaging study recently conducted by our group was a difference between the sexes in the relationship between intracranial volume and height (P. C. Nopoulos, M. Flaum, and N. C. Andreasen, "Gender Differences in Brain Morphology: Regional Measures, Tissue Composition, and Surface Anatomy," April 1999 [unpublished study]). As described previously (see subsection above titled "Sex Differences in Structural Morphology"), MRI was used to evaluate the brain morphology of 42 healthy females matched with 42 healthy males by age and IQ. The relationship between height (in centimeters [cm]) and cerebral tissue volume (in cubic centimeters [cc]) was evaluated with Pearson correlation coefficients and showed a strong positive correlation for the females ($r = 0.43$, $P = .003$). For the male subjects, however, there was no significant relationship ($r = -0.02$, $P = .867$). The two correlations were found to be statistically different ($z = 2.16$, $P = .03$) (see Figure 1–2). These findings suggest that the factors that govern overall body growth (resulting in height) are not closely related to or regulated by the factors that determine brain growth in men. On the other hand, for women, overall body size does to some degree determine overall brain size.

Although somewhat unexpected, our findings are very similar to those from an MRI study on the striatum. Raz et al. (1992) found that the volume of the caudate nucleus was positively correlated with skull size ($r = 0.46$, $P < .025$) in females but showed a nonsignificant trend in the opposite direction in males ($r = -0.22$ [not

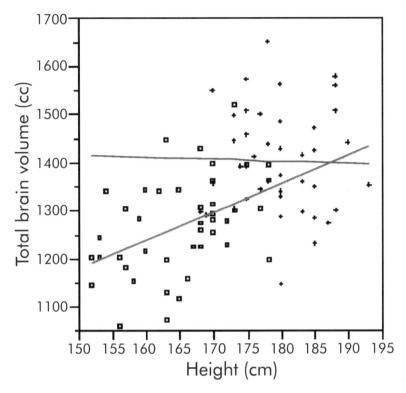

Figure 1–2. Relationship between height and total brain volume. □ = Female *(green line)*; Pearson correlation $r = 0.43$ ($P = .003$). ✛ = Male *(red line)*; Pearson correlation $r = -0.02$ ($P = .867$).

significant]). The pattern is the same for cerebral tissue volume (P. C. Nopoulos, M. Flaum, and N. C. Andreasen, "Gender Differences in Brain Morphology: Regional Measures, Tissue Composition, and Surface Anatomy," April 1999 [unpublished study]) as it is for caudate nucleus volume (Raz et al. 1992): there is a positive correlation in females, but not in males, between brain/caudate volume and height/skull size. Although it is difficult to speculate on the functional interpretation of these findings, it appears that substructures of the male brain appear to grow independently of overall skull size, similar to the previously discussed finding that in males the growth of the entire cerebrum is independent of overall height. In females, however, the growth of the cerebrum and of substructures such as the caudate is more closely linked to overall body and skull size.

Sex Differences in Lateralization

Structural Lateralization

Sex differences in cerebral lateralization were first reported more than 100 years ago in a postmortem gross anatomy study, in which female brains exhibited greater symmetry with regard to weights of the left and right hemispheres. Several authors have postulated that circulating testosterone levels in utero influence the developing brain by either promoting the growth of the right hemisphere or delaying the development of the left hemisphere (Bear et al. 1986). However, throughout the mid-1900s, studies of lateralization yielded inconsistent findings, and by the 1960s, researchers were describing the morphometric literature as lacking conclusive evidence for any significant sex differences in cerebral lateralization. The findings of recent MRI studies are consonant with this assessment, as most of these studies have failed to find a significant interaction between sex and hemispheric asymmetry in either the child/adolescent brain (Giedd et al. 1996; Reiss et al. 1996) or the adult brain (Coffey et al. 1998; Murphy et al. 1996). An exception to this lack of findings supporting gender differences in cerebral lateralization was a study by Bear et al. (1986) that found greater degrees of frontal and occipital asymmetries in men than in women.

Although overall cerebral asymmetries may not vary by sex, regional asymmetries may. A 1975 study that examined 100 postmortem adult brains reported that the brains that showed reversals of the usual pattern of planum temporale asymmetry (left larger than right) were much more likely to be female. This pattern was also found in a sample of 100 postmortem infant brains (Wada et al. 1975). This finding in adults was recently replicated in an MRI study that found nonsignificant left–right differences in the planum temporale area in females, but significant left–right differences in males (left larger than right). These data support the notion of reduced asymmetry among females (Kulynych et al. 1994).

Another main focus in studies of sex differences in the brain with regard to lateralization involves communication between the two sides of the brain mediated through the corpus callosum. The "saga" of alleged sex differences in the size and/or shape of the corpus callosum is an interesting piece of science history. More than any other aspect of brain morphology, the corpus callosum is most often cited as an example of sex differences in brain morphology. Specifically, there appears to be a widely held belief that differences exist in the shape of the splenium of the corpus callosum, with the splenium in females having a more "bulbous" shape than that in males. This claim is based on a small postmortem study (nine males and five females) by de Lacoste-Utamsing and Holloway (1982). Despite numerous attempts in subsequent studies, the finding was never replicated, with the exception of an extension and replication study done by the original authors (Holloway and de Lacoste 1986) and a study by Allen et al. (1991) using the de Lacoste method. The absence of a sex difference in the size/shape of the corpus callosum was confirmed in a recent meta-analysis by Bishop and Wahlsten (1997) of 49 studies published since 1980. This analysis detected no significant sex differences in the size or shape of the splenium of the corpus callosum, regardless of whether an appropriate adjustment was made for brain size using ANCOVA or linear regression. In their review, Bishop and Wahlsten note that recent MRI studies do, however, confirm the early (prior to 1910) postmortem findings of larger average brain size and overall corpus callosum size in males.

Functional Lateralization

In addition to structural asymmetries between the hemispheres, the brain is known to have functional asymmetry in its representation of cognitive processes. For example, receptive and expressive aspects of language are predominantly represented in, and/or are more efficiently processed by, the left hemisphere. The findings of several studies of cerebral lateralization differences between the sexes suggest that the male brain is functionally organized in a more asymmetrical fashion than the female brain, which implies that females have more bilateral function. This notion is supported by studies performed in stroke patients, which show that after a left-hemisphere stroke, men are more likely than women to have a pervasive and lasting language disorder; this finding suggests that women have more bilateral function for language than do men (McGlone 1980). A recent study (Shaywitz et al. 1995) used fMRI to study asymmetries in the brains of men and women. Male and female subjects were asked to perform a variety of language tasks that focused on non-production aspects of language such as phonological processing. Brain activation in males was shown to be lateralized to the left frontal regions, but in females the pattern of activation was *bilateral* in the frontal regions (Shaywitz et al. 1995). Additionally, a study evaluating magnetoencephalographic auditory evoked field differences between the sexes found a sex-based difference in right superior temporal gyrus functional anatomy, with evidence of greater hemispheric lateralization in men compared with women (Reite et al. 1995).

However, a recent PET study that evaluated speech production tasks in men and women found no significant sex differences (Buckner et al. 1995), and an fMRI study evaluating a verbal fluency task showed no gross differences in the pattern of activation between male and female subjects (Schlosser et al. 1998). These two studies suggest that if any gender differences exist in the brain's functional organization for language, they may involve only very specific aspects of language such as phonological processing.

Regardless of differences in laterality of brain morphology or function between the sexes, some have argued that there are important sex differences in the relationship between structure and function. An MRI study by Willerman et al. (1992) found that in men, a larger left hemisphere relative to the right predicted better verbal than nonverbal ability, yet a larger left hemisphere predicted relatively better nonverbal than verbal ability in women. The authors concluded that the reversed hemisphere size–ability relationships in the women suggest that the neural substrate governing nonverbal problem solving is distributed over both hemispheres, which again lends partial support to the notion that cognitive ability in females may be more bilateral than that in males.

Sex Differences in Brain Activity

Functional Studies of Brain Blood
Flow and Glucose Metabolism

Several groups using functional neuroimaging methods have reported that females have higher generalized cerebral blood flow than do males (for a review, see R. E. Gur and R. C. Gur 1990). The basis for the higher blood flow in females is not entirely clear. Some have suggested that systemic factors such as the effect of circulating estrogen may play a role, although no studies have assessed this hypothesis directly. Other possible factors include heart rate, pulse pressure, and cardiac index, all of which lead to higher body/brain blood flow and are higher in females than in males. Finally, as previously mentioned, Schlaepfer et al. (1995) have suggested that women's higher cerebral blood flow may be due to their increased gray-matter volumes in comparison with men. Although this is an interesting notion, the increases in cerebral blood flow found in women have typically been global, whereas the increase in gray-matter volume reported in the Schlaepfer et al. article was regional only.

In contrast to the studies that have shown increases in cerebral blood flow in women, the findings for increases in glucose metabolism are not as consistent. Although Baxter et al. (1987) and Yoshii et al. (1988) both reported higher brain glucose metabolism in females than in males, and Andreason et al. (1993) showed only a trend ($P = .06$, one tailed) for higher metabolism in females, other studies have found no sex differences (Azari et al. 1992; R. C. Gur et al. 1995; Miura et al. 1990). Some authors have suggested that the higher rate of metabolism in women reported by some studies is related to women's smaller volume of brain tissue. Hatazawa et al. (1987) used PET to study blood glucose utilization and found that whereas women's brains were 9% smaller than men's brains, brain metabolism in women was 9% higher than that in men. The authors also found that metabolic rates in the brain are inversely proportional to brain size, regardless of sex. Therefore, Hatazawa and colleagues concluded that since women's brain size is reduced by the same amount as their metabolic rate is increased in relation to men's, the sex differences in metabolic rate would most likely disappear after adjustment for brain size.

Functional Studies of The Resting State

In a PET study by R. C. Gur et al. (1995), sex differences in regional distribution of cerebral glucose metabolism were evaluated during a resting state. Men were found to have higher metabolism than women in temporolimbic regions and the cerebellum. Conversely, women had higher metabolism than men in the cingulate region, one of the more complex components of the limbic system that regulates emotional processes. The authors concluded that these findings supported a neurobiological explanation of some sex differences in behavior, such as emotional processing, given that women tend to feel and express emotions more frequently and more intensely than men. In addition, an MRI study by Paus et al. (1996) found a structural corollary to the functional imaging results of R. C. Gur et al. (1995), reporting that females had significantly higher cingulate gyrus volumes compared with males.

A more recent study by Volkow et al. (1997) found no sex differences in whole-brain metabolism. However, women were found to have consistent increases in cerebellar metabolism. This finding is in contrast to that of the R. C. Gur et al. (1995) study, which found higher cerebellar metabolism in men, although the fact that the study populations of the two investigations differed significantly in age may account for their different results. Moreover, there is mounting evidence that the cerebellum is involved in emotional (Berman et al. 1974) and cognitive skills (Andreasen et al. 1995), including language (Leiner et al. 1993), in addition to its well-known involvement in motor coordination. This highlights once again the precept that important sex differences in brain function need not be accompanied by significant differences in brain structure.

The Aging Brain

The effects of aging on the brain, like those of neurodevelopment and maturation, are poorly understood. Moreover, only a small number of imaging studies have examined the effects of sex on brain aging in normal populations. In one of the earliest studies to report sex differences in the aging process, our group found that although ventricular size increased dramatically over time in men beginning around the age of 40, this phenomenon was delayed by a full decade for women (Andreasen et al. 1990). Since that study, the literature has been mostly consistent in its findings that males show greater aging changes than do females. Although study findings regarding sex-specific effects of aging on brain regions are quite inconsistent, three studies have indicated that men have greater age-related volume loss in the temporal lobe than do women, and at least two studies have found men to also have greater age-related volume loss in the frontal lobes. R. C. Gur et al. (1991) found a lateralized aging effect, with the left hemisphere decreasing in volume over time more robustly for men than for women.

The neurobiological basis for the sexual dimorphism in brain aging is not known, although the "usual suspects" of neuroendocrinological differences between the sexes have been postulated. Also important is the higher incidence of risk factors for vascular pathology in men, which may account for tissue loss due to cerebral microvascular disease. Finally, it is known from the neurodevelopmental literature that the pace of cerebral development is much slower in males than in females and that brain growth is completed at a younger age in females than in males. It is also thought that the slower growth rate in the male brain imparts a serious vulnerability, making it more susceptible to environmental adversity in the perinatal period. This slower growth rate may also be a factor in the higher prevalence of neuropsychiatric disorders in males compared with females (see next section). Therefore, with regard to the aging process, it has been postulated that structures that develop later may in some way be more susceptible to degeneration with aging.

Relationship Between Sexual Dimorphism in the Brain and Psychopathology

As mentioned in the introduction to this chapter, one of the reasons for the increased interest in the effects of gender on brain morphology is the need to better evaluate the interaction between sex differences in the brain and disease pathology. Almost all neuropsychiatric disorders have significant sex differences in presentation, course, severity, and, often, treatment response. Most childhood neurodevelopmental syndromes—such as mental retardation, learning disorders, communication disorders, autism, attention-deficit/hyperactivity disorder, and enuresis—occur more often in males than in females (American Psychiatric Association 1994). It is important to note that these are not exclusively male disorders; they do occur in females, but less frequently and possibly to a less severe extent. For example, severe mental retardation is more common in males (Broman et al. 1987). In regard to adult psychopathology, lifetime prevalence is higher in women compared with men for panic disorder, phobic disorder, somatization disorder, and mood disorders (Robins and Regier 1991). For schizophrenia, there is some debate as to whether there is a difference in prevalence between the sexes, though it is well documented that age at onset (Lewine 1988), premorbid adjustment (Zigler et al. 1979), symptom profile (Castle and Murray 1991), medication response, and outcome (Seeman 1986) are significantly different for men and women with this illness. In the elderly population, Alzheimer's disease appears to be more common among women (Gao et al. 1998), and estrogen replacement may possibly have both a preventive and a treatment role. To understand fully the interaction between sexual dimorphism in the brain and disease pathology, we must first elucidate each of these components independently. Without a doubt, we are far from having a good understanding of sex differences in the normal brain, and the mysteries of pathoetiologies of neuropsychiatric illnesses loom large. Therefore, this is a daunting task indeed. In the following subsections we examine the possible relationships between sex differences in brain structure/function and disease pathology by reviewing studies of schizophrenia and depression.

Schizophrenia

Over the last several years, accumulating evidence indicates that the etiology of schizophrenia is neurodevelopmental (Waddington and Buckley 1996). As mentioned earlier in this chapter, there is considerable evidence to support phenomenological differences between men and women in schizophrenia. Males display a more severe illness with an earlier age at onset, poorer premorbid function, more negative symptoms, and poorer overall outcome. Sex differences in early brain development may be at the root of this disparity.

In early development, the pace of cerebral development is slower in males than in females (Kretschmann et al. 1979). This relative slowness may cause the brain of the male infant to be more vulnerable to a variety of problems, such as environmental insults or developmental disease pathology. For instance, low-birth-weight males are more likely than their female counterparts to develop intra- and periventricular hemorrhage and to experience long-term adverse neurological deficits as a result (Amato et al. 1987). Also, as previously mentioned, the prevalence of many neurodevelopmental disorders, such as autism, language disorders, and attention-deficit/hyperactivity disorder is higher in males than in females. With regard to schizophrenia, sex differences in disease-related changes in brain morphology are consonant with this theme. That is, of the studies that have evaluated sex differences in brain morphology in patients with schizophrenia, most have found males to have more severe structural abnormalities than females (Nopoulos et al. 1997a). A study conducted in our center found that developmental brain anomalies such as enlarged cavum septi pellucidi are more frequent in patients with schizophrenia, and particularly male patients (Nopoulos et al. 1997b). In another study from our center, brain morphology was evaluated in a group of 40 male patients and 40 female patients matched by age and gender to healthy control subjects. The results showed that the difference in brain morphology between the sexes was a matter of severity rather than of pattern—that is, the brains of females with schizophrenia manifested the same pattern of abnormalities seen in males, but to a lesser degree. In particular, the finding of enlarged ventricles in schizophrenia appears to be a predominantly male phenomenon (Nopoulos et al. 1997a).

Another study of brain morphology in schizophrenia indicated important sex differences of a different type. Cowell et al. (1996) found that in men with schizophrenia, smaller frontal lobe size was associated with more severe disorganization. In contrast, in women, larger frontal lobe volume was associated with greater severity of disorganization and "suspicion–hostility." This study highlights the importance of looking beyond simple structural differences between the sexes to investigate differences in the relationships between brain function and brain structure.

Depression

The incidence of depression among women is as much as four times that of men, with epidemiological studies reporting lifetime rates of 20%–25% in women as compared with 7%–12% in men (Depression Guideline Panel 1993). In a study by George et al. (1996), functional imaging with PET was used to evaluate cerebral blood flow during transient self-induced states of sadness or happiness. The study included 10 men and 10 age-matched women who were scanned at rest and during happy, sad, and neutral states self-induced by recalling affect-appropriate life events and looking at happy, sad, or neutral human faces. Women activated a significantly wider portion of their limbic systems than did men during transient sadness, despite similar self-reported changes in mood. Moreover, one of the areas with greater activation in women compared with men during induced sadness was the mesial prefrontal cortex, an area that has been shown to be hypoactive in patients with depression (George et al. 1993). Although they represent only indirect evidence, these findings suggest that women may have some vulnerability to depression based on differential functioning of the limbic system.

Serotonin metabolism in the brain has been shown to be important in the pathophysiology of depression, as demonstrated by the effectiveness of serotonin reuptake inhibitors in the treatment of depression. In a very interesting study using PET, Nishizawa et al. (1997) were able to measure the rates of serotonin synthesis in the human brain. Unlike indolamine levels, which were uniform throughout the brain, serotonin levels were found to vary greatly in different brain areas. Moreover, the mean rate of serotonin synthesis in normal males was found to be 52% higher than that in normal females. This sex difference is quite robust, and because serotonin has direct relevance to the pathophysiology of depression, these findings strongly support the notion that the female brain has a neurochemical liability to mood disorders.

Summary

In many respects, the male brain and the female brain are very similar indeed. Nevertheless, against the background of similarity, the structure of the human brain does have some important differences between the sexes. Sexual dimorphism in the human brain has been reported not only at a gross level but also at the level of regions, at the level of tissue composition of regions, and—possibly most importantly—at the level of the relationships between structure and function.

Nonetheless, it is one thing to identify biological substrates that may account for sex differences in emotion and cognition, but quite another to elucidate the etiologies of these differences. Although these types of findings are very interesting, they do not shed light on the age-old question of whether the between-sex differences in the brain are "hardwired" or are modeled and molded within a substrate (the brain) that is heavily influenced by its environment.

References

Abramovich D, Rowe P: Foetal plasma testosterone levels at mid-pregnancy and at term: relationship to foetal sex. J Endocrinol 56: 621–622, 1973

Allen L, Richey M, Chai Y, et al: Sex differences in the corpus callosum of the living human being. J Neurosci 11:933–942, 1991

Amato M, Howald H, von Muralt G: Fetal sex and distribution of peri-ventricular hemorrhage in preterm infants. European Journal of Neurology 27:20–23, 1987

American Psychiatric Association: Diagnostic and Statistical Manual of Mental Disorders, 4th Edition. Washington, DC, American Psychiatric Association, 1994

Andreasen NC, Swayze V, Flaum M, et al: Ventricular enlargement in schizophrenia evaluated with CT scanning: effects of gender, age, and stage of illness. Arch Gen Psychiatry 47:1054–1059, 1990

Andreasen NCA, Flashman L, Flaum M, et al: Regional brain abnormalities in schizophrenia measured with magnetic resonance imaging. JAMA 272:1763–1769, 1994

Andreasen NC, O'Leary DS, Arndt S, et al: Short-term and long-term verbal memory: a positron emission tomography study. Proc Natl Acad Sci U S A 92:5111–5115, 1995

Andreason PJ, Zametkin AJ, Guo AC, et al: Gender-related differences in regional cerebral glucose metabolism in normal volunteers. Psychiatry Res 51:175–183, 1993

Azari NP, Rapoport SE, Grady CL, et al: Gender differences in correlations of cerebral glucose metabolic rates in young adult normal humans. Brain Res 574:198–208, 1992

Baxter LR, Mazziotta JC, Phelps ME, et al: Cerebral glucose metabolic rates. Psychiatry Res 21:237–245, 1987

Bear D, Schiff D, Saver J, et al: Quantitative analysis of cerebral asymmetries. Arch Neurol 43:598–603, 1986

Benes FM, Turtle M, Khan Y, et al: Myelination of a key relay zone in the hippocampal formation occurs in the human brain during childhood, adolescence, and adulthood. Arch Gen Psychiatry 51:477–484, 1994

Berman AJ, Berman D, Prescott JW: The effect of cerebellar lesions on emotional behavior in the rhesus monkey, in The Cerebellum, Epilepsy, and Behavior. Edited by Cooper IS, Riklan N, Snider RS. New York, Plenum, 1974, pp 277–284

Bishop KM, Wahlsten D: Sex differences in the human corpus callosum: myth or reality? Neurosci Biobehav Rev 21:581–601, 1997

Blinkow S, Glezer I: The Human Brain in Figures and Tables: A Quantitative Handbook. New York, Basic Books, 1968

Broman S, Nichols PL, Shaughnessy P, et al: Retardation in Young Children: A Developmental Study of Cognitive Deficit. Hillsdale, NJ, Lawrence Erlbaum, 1987

Buckner RL, Raichle MR, Petersen SE: Dissociation of human prefrontal cortical areas across different speech production tasks and gender groups. J Neurophysiol 74:2163–2173, 1995

Carlson M, Earls F, Todd RD: The importance of regressive changes in the development of the nervous system: towards a neurobiological theory of child development. Psychiatric Developments 1(6):1–22, 1988

Castle D, Murray R: The neurodevelopmental basis of sex differences in schizophrenia. Psychol Med 21:565–575, 1991

Caviness VS, Kennedy DN, Richelme C, et al: The human brain age 7–11 years: a volumetric analysis based on magnetic resonance images. Cereb Cortex 6:726–736, 1996

Coffey CE, Lucke JF, Saxton JA, et al: Sex differences in brain aging. Arch Neurol 55:169–179, 1998

Cowell PE, Kostianovsky DJ, Gur RC, et al: Sex differences in neuroanatomical and clinical correlations in schizophrenia. Am J Psychiatry 153:799–805, 1996

Dekaban A, Sadowski D: Changes in brain weights during the span of human life: relation of brain weights to body heights and body weight. Ann Neurol 44:345–356, 1978

de Lacoste-Utamsing C, Holloway RL: Sexual dimorphism in the human corpus callosum. Science 216:1431–1432, 1982

Depression Guideline Panel: Depression in Primary Care, Vol 1: Detection and Diagnosis. Rockville, MD, U.S. Department of Health and Human Services, 1993

Ehrhardt A, Meyer-Bahlburg H, Rosen L, et al: Sexual orientation after prenatal exposure to exogenous estrogen. Arch Sex Behav 14:57–77, 1985

Feinberg I: Schizophrenia: caused by a fault in programmed synaptic elimination during adolescence? J Psychiatr Res 17:319–334, 1982

Feldman JF, Brody N, Miller SA: Sex differences in non-elicited neonatal behaviors. Merrill Palmer Quarterly 26(1):63–73, 1980

Filipek R, Richelme C, Kennedy D, et al: The young adult human brain: an MRI-based morphometric analysis. Cereb Cortex 4:344–360, 1994

Gao S, Hendrie HC, Hall KS, et al: The relationships between age, sex, and the incidence of dementia and Alzheimer disease. Arch Gen Psychiatry 55:809–815, 1998

George MS, Ketter TA, Post RM: SPECT and PET imaging in mood disorders. J Clin Psychiatry 64:6–13, 1993

George MS, Ketter TA, Parekh PI, et al: Gender differences in regional cerebral blood flow during transient self-induced sadness or happiness. Biol Psychiatry 40:859–871, 1996

Geschwind NW, Galaburda AM: Cerebral lateralization: biological mechanisms, associations and pathology. Arch Neurol 42:428–552, 1985

Ghez C: The cerebellum, in Principles of Neural Science. Edited by Kandel E, Schwartz J, Jessel T. Norwalk, CT, Appleton & Lange, 1991, pp 626–646

Giedd J, Snell J, Lange N, et al: Quantitative magnetic resonance imaging of human brain development: ages 4–18. Cereb Cortex 6:551–560, 1996

Grattan MP, De Vos E, Levy J, et al: Asymmetric action in the human newborn: sex differences in patterns of organization. Child Dev 63: 273–289, 1992

Gur RC, Mozley PD, Resnick SM, et al: Gender differences in age effect on brain atrophy measured by magnetic resonance imaging. Proc Natl Acad Sci U S A 88:2845–2849, 1991

Gur RC, Mozley LH, Mozley PD, et al: Sex differences in regional cerebral glucose metabolism during a resting state. Science 267:528–531, 1995

Gur RE, Gur RC: Gender differences in regional cerebral blood flow. Schizophr Bull 16:247–254, 1990

Hamburger V: Trophic interactions in neurogenesis: a personal historical account. Annu Rev Neurosci 3:269–278, 1980

Hatazawa J, Brooks RA, Di Chiro G, et al: Global cerebral glucose utilization is independent of brain size: a PET study. J Comput Assist Tomogr 11:571–576, 1987

Hittelman JH, Dickes R: Sex differences in neonatal eye contact time. Merrill Palmer Quarterly 25(3):171–184, 1979

Ho K-C, Roessmann U, Straumfjord JV, et al: Analysis of brain weight, I: adult brain weight in relation to sex, race, and age. Arch Pathol Lab Med 104:635–639, 1980

Holloway RL, de Lacoste MC: Sexual dimorphism in the human corpus callosum: an extension and replication study. Human Neurobiology 5:87–91, 1986

Jacklin CN, Snow ME, Maccoby EE: Tactile sensitivity and muscle strength in newborn boys and girls. Infant Behavior and Development 4:261–268, 1981

Jernigan TL, Tallal P: Late childhood changes in brain morphology observable with MRI. Dev Med Child Neurol 32:379–385, 1990

Kawata M: Roles of steroid hormones and their receptors in structural organization in the nervous system. Neurosci Res 24:1–46, 1995

Keshavan MS, Anderson S, Pettegrew JW: Is schizophrenia due to excessive synaptic pruning in the prefrontal cortex? The Feinberg hypothesis revisited. J Psychiatr Res 28:239–265, 1994

Korner AF: Sex differences in newborns with special reference to differences in the organization of oral behavior. J Child Psychol Psychiatry 14:19–29, 1973

Kretschmann HJ, Schleicher A, Wingert F, et al: Human brain growth in the 19th and 20th century. J Neurol Sci 40:169–188, 1979

Kulynych J, Vladar K, Jones D, et al: Gender differences in the normal lateralization of the supratemporal cortex: MRI surface-rendering morphometry of Heschl's gyrus and the planum temporale. Cereb Cortex 4:107–118, 1994

Leiner HC, Leiner AL, Dow RS: Cognitive and language skills of the human cerebellum. Trends Neurosci 16:444–447, 1993

Lewine RJ: Gender and schizophrenia, in Handbook of Schizophrenia: Nosology, Epidemiology, and Genetics. Edited by Tsuang MT, Simpson J. Amsterdam, Elsevier Science, 1988, pp 379–398

MacLusky NJ, Naftolin F: Sexual differentiation of the central nervous system. Science 211:1294–1302, 1981

Masica D, Money J, Ehrhardt A, et al: IQ, fetal sex hormones and cognitive patterns: studies in the testicular feminizing syndrome of androgen insensitivity. Johns Hopkins Medical Journal 124:34–43, 1969

McGlone J: Sex differences in human brain asymmetry: a critical survey. Behav Brain Sci 3:215–63, 1980

Miura S, Schapiro M, Grady C, et al: Effect of gender on glucose utilization rates in healthy humans: a positron emission tomography study. J Neurosci Res 4:500–504, 1990

Murphy DGM, DeCarli C, McIntosh AR, et al: Sex differences in human brain morphometry and metabolism: an in vivo quantitative magnetic resonance imaging and positron emission tomography study of the effect of aging. Arch Gen Psychiatry 53:585–594, 1996

Nishizawa S, Benkelfat C, Young SN, et al: Differences between males and females in rates of serotonin synthesis in human brain. Proc Natl Acad Sci U S A 94:5308–5313, 1997

Nopoulos PC, Flaum M, Andreasen NC: Sex differences in brain morphology in schizophrenia. Am J Psychiatry 154:1648–1654, 1997a

Nopoulos P, Swayze V, Flaum M, et al: Cavum septi pellucidi in normals and patients with schizophrenia as detected by MRI. Biol Psychiatry 41:1102–1108, 1997b

Passe TJ, Rafagopalan P, Tupler LA, et al: Age and sex effects on brain morphology. Prog Neuropsychopharmacol Biol Psychiatry 21:1231–1237, 1997

Paus T, Otaky M, Caramanos Z, et al: In vivo morphometry of the intrasulcal gray matter in the human cingulate, paracingulate, and superior-rostral sulci: hemispheric asymmetries, gender differences, and probability maps. J Comp Neurol 376:664–673, 1996

Pfefferbaum A, Mathalon DH, Sullivan EV, et al: A quantitative magnetic resonance imaging study of changes in brain morphology from infancy to late adulthood. Arch Neurol 51:874–887, 1994

Pilgrim C, Hutchinson JB: Developmental regulation of sex differences in the brain: can the role of gonadal steroids be redefined? Neuroscience 60:843–855, 1994

Purves D, Lichtman JW: Principles of Neural Development. Sunderland, MA, Sinauer Associates, 1985

Raz N, Torres IJ, Spencer WD, et al: Age-related regional differences in cerebellar vermis observed in vivo. Arch Neurol 49:412–416, 1992

Reinisch J, Gandelman R, Spiegel F: Prenatal gonadal steroidal influences on gender-related behavior, in Progress in Brain Research: Sex Differences in the Brain. Edited by DeVried G, De Brui J, Uylings H, et al. Amsterdam, Elsevier, 1979, pp 407–416

Reiss AL, Abrams MT, Singer HS, et al: Brain development, gender and IQ in children: a volumetric imaging study. Brain 119:1763–1774, 1996

Reite M, Sheeder J, Teale P, et al: MEG-based brain laterality: sex differences in normal adults. Neuropsychologica 33:1607–1616, 1995

Resnick SM, Berenbaum SA, Gottesman II, et al: Early hormonal influences on cognitive functioning in congenital adrenal hyperplasia. Dev Psychol 22:191–198, 1986

Restak R: The Brain: The Last Frontier. New York, Doubleday, 1979

Robins LM, Reiger DA: Psychiatric Disorders in America. New York, Free Press, 1991

Schlaepfer TE, Harris GJ, Tien AY, et al: Structural differences in the cerebral cortex of healthy female and male subjects: a magnetic resonance imaging study. Psychiatry Res: Neuroimaging 61:129–135, 1995

Schlosser R, Hutchinson M, Joseffer S, et al: Functional magnetic resonance imaging of human brain activity in a verbal fluency task. J Neurol Neurosurg Psychiatry 64:492–498, 1998

Seeman MV: Current outcome in schizophrenia: women vs. men. Acta Psychiatr Scand 73:609–617, 1986

Shaywitz B, Shaywitz S, Pugh K, et al: Sex differences in the functional organization of the brain for language. Nature 373:607–609, 1995

Talairach J, Tournoux P: Co-Planar Stereotaxic Atlas of the Human Brain. New York, Thieme Medical Publishers, 1988

Volkow ND, Wang GJ, Fowler JS, et al: Gender differences in cerebellar metabolism: test-retest reproducibility. Am J Psychiatry 154:119–121, 1997

Wada JA, Clarke R, Hamm A: Cerebral hemisphere asymmetry in humans: cortical speech zones in 100 adult and 100 infant brains. Arch Neurol 32:239–246, 1975

Waddington JL, Buckley P (eds): The Neurodevelopmental Basis of Schizophrenia. Austin, TX, RG Landes, 1996

Willerman L, Schultz R, Rutledge JN, et al: Hemisphere size asymmetry predicts relative verbal and nonverbal intelligence differently in the sexes: an MRI study of structure-function relations. Intelligence 16:315–328, 1992

Yoshii F, Barker WW, Chang JY: Sensitivity of cerebral glucose metabolism to age, gender, brain volume, brain atrophy and cerebrovascular risk factors. J Cereb Blood Flow Metab 8:654–661, 1988

Zigler E, Glick M, Marsh A: Premorbid social competence and outcome among schizophrenic and nonschizophrenic patients. J Nerv Ment Dis 167:478–483, 1979

Chapter 2

Women, Stress, and Depression: Sex Differences in Hypothalamic-Pituitary-Adrenal Axis Regulation

Elizabeth Young, M.D., and
Ania Korszun, M.D., Ph.D.

Depression is a multifactorial disorder in which adaptation to stressors undoubtedly plays a crucial role. Although genetic vulnerability is critical to the development of depression, in the absence of environmental stressors, the incidence of depressive disorders is very low (Kendler et al. 1995), and in approximately 75% of cases of depression there is a precipitating life event (Brown and Harris 1978; Frank et al. 1994). An understanding of the pathoetiology of depression must address the observed relationship between stress and depression while also providing an explanation for the high preponderance of women in the population of those with depressive disorders. Thus, the relationship among gender, depression, and stress—and, in particular, sex differences in the stress hormone response—is an intriguing and fruitful area of research.

Living organisms survive by maintaining a complex dynamic equilibrium, or *homeostasis*, that is constantly challenged by intrinsic or extrinsic stressors. These stressors set in motion responses aimed at preserving homeostasis, including activation of the hypothalamic-pituitary-adrenal (HPA) axis. A hormonal cascade is initiated by release of corticotropin-releasing hormone (CRH), which triggers the release of adrenocorticotropic hormone (ACTH) from the anterior pituitary corticotrope, which in turn triggers the release of adrenal glucocorticoids. The stress response is turned off by glucocorticoid feedback at brain and pituitary sites (Figure 2–1). As detailed later in this chapter, there is evidence in both rats and humans that the stress response is sexually dimorphic, and our studies in rats and humans have suggested that gonadal steroids play an important role in modulating the HPA axis, acting particularly on sensitivity to glucocorticoid negative feedback (Young et al. 1993). Gonadal steroids may influence the HPA axis feedback mechanisms through effects on glucocorticoid receptors, on brain CRH systems, or on pituitary responsiveness to CRH.

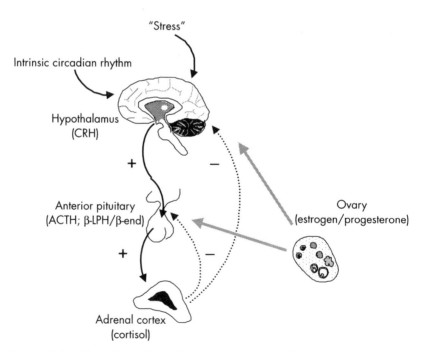

Figure 2–1. Overview of hypothalamic-pituitary-adrenal (HPA) axis function. ACTH = adrenocorticotropic hormone; β-LPH/β-end = β-lipotropin and β-endorphin; CRH = corticotropin-releasing hormone.

HPA Axis Regulation

Glucocorticoids act via multiple mechanisms, at several sites, to inhibit their own release. At the pituitary level, glucocorticoids exert direct effects on the ACTH precursor prohormone proopiomelanocorticotropin (POMC), influencing gene transcription, POMC messenger RNA (mRNA) levels, and subsequent ACTH peptide stores in primary pituitary cell cultures in vitro (Birnberg et al. 1982, 1983; Roberts et al. 1979; Schachter et al. 1982). These effects involve the classic glucocorticoid receptor (GR Type II), which binds glucocorticoids, is translocated to the nucleus, and binds to sites on the DNA (Schachter et al. 1982). Studies have demonstrated that glucocorticoids interact with the CRH receptors in the anterior pituitary, acutely inhibiting the binding of CRH to its receptors and chronically decreasing CRH receptor numbers (Childs et al. 1986; Schwartz et al. 1986). Such direct effects of glucocorticoids on CRH receptors may account for some of the inhibitory action of glucocorticoids on ACTH release in vitro.

In addition to pituitary sites of action, glucocorticoids act at brain sites to modulate HPA axis activity. Early work by McEwen and colleagues (1968) demonstrated high-affinity sites for corticosterone in the hippocampus of adrenalectomized rats injected in vivo with radiolabeled steroids. These receptors were difficult to demonstrate in nonadrenalectomized rats, presumably because these sites were saturated under resting conditions (McEwen et al. 1970). The receptors were not labeled by [^{3}H]dexamethasone, a finding suggesting the existence of multiple types of glucocorticoid receptors (de Kloet et al. 1975). The observation of receptor heterogeneity was expanded upon by de Kloet and colleagues, who subsequently demonstrated the existence of two glucocorticoid receptor types: mineralocorticoid receptors, which have a particularly high affinity for the glucocorticoid *corticosterone*, and glucocorticoid receptors, which preferentially bind dexamethasone (Reul and de Kloet 1985). Glucocorticoid receptors are widely distributed throughout the brain, whereas mineralocorticoid receptors exist predominantly in the hippocampus. In addition to the glucocorticoids' action at the pituitary and hypothalamus, there is strong evidence from animal experiments that the hippocampus is the main glucocorticoid feedback site in the brain.

The importance of hippocampal steroid receptors in feedback regulation of stress has been demonstrated in several studies (Sapolsky et al. 1986). Removal of the hippocampus leads to an increase in anterior pituitary secretion of β-endorphin in plasma, an increase in CRH mRNA in the paraventricular nucleus of the hypothalamus (PVN), and a limited induction of vasopressin mRNA in parvocellular neurons of the PVN (Herman et al. 1989). In a formulation that may be relevant to depressive disorders, Sapolsky and colleagues (1986) have proposed the glucocorticoid cascade hypothesis, a model that describes the effects of chronic stress on hippocampal neurons. According to this model, repeated stress—or chronic glucocorticoid administration—downregulates hippocampal steroid receptors, but not hypothalamic or pituitary receptors (Sapolsky et al. 1986; Young and Vazquez 1996). Animals with downregulated hippocampal glucocorticoid receptors exhibit delays in the turnoff of the glucocorticoid response to stress and demonstrate decreased sensitivity to glucocorticoid fast feedback (Young and Vazquez 1996). This decrease in glucocorticoid receptors and insensitivity to negative feedback leads to prolonged hypercortisolism, which eventually can result in atrophy of hippocampal neurons and further glucocorticoid hypersecretion. Glucocorticoid hypersecretion and hippocampal neuronal atrophy are most pronounced in aged rats, a situation analogous to that reported in human depression, in which there is a higher incidence of HPA axis feedback abnormalities in elderly individuals (Akil et al. 1993; Halbreich et al. 1984; Lewis et al. 1984; Young et al. 1995).

Sex Differences in HPA Axis Regulation: Studies in Patients With Depression

Abnormalities of the HPA axis, as manifested by hypercortisolemia and disruption of the circadian rhythm of cortisol secretion, are well-established phenomena in depression (Carroll et al. 1976; Sachar et al. 1973). In addition, depressed patients are less likely than control subjects to suppress ACTH and cortisol secretion after receiving dexamethasone (Sachar et al. 1973). Our group has demonstrated sex differences in HPA axis function in depressed patients. These data are reviewed in this section, together with the evidence for similar sex differences both in animals and in humans without mood disorders (see Table 2–1). This sexual dimorphism of the stress response has important implications for our current understanding of the increased susceptibility of women to depression and other psychiatric disorders, particularly at certain times during the reproductive life cycle.

Morning and Evening Cortisol Hypersecretion

Data from several studies indicate that, among depressed patients, women are more likely than men to have abnormalities in HPA axis regulation. For example, we measured baseline cortisol secretion in the morning in 16 depressed patients and 16 age- and sex-matched control patients and found predictably increased cortisol secretion in the group as a whole (Young et al. 1991). However, there were also clear sex differences: male patients and their matched control subjects had similar plasma cortisol concentrations, whereas female depressed patients demonstrated significantly higher mean plasma cortisol concentrations (11.3 ± 0.9 μg/dL) than did their matched controls (8.1 ± 0.95 μg/dL; significant by a two-tailed t test, $P = .033$). This finding suggests that the generally reported hypercortisolemia of depression may be a result of the fact that samples of depressed patients usually include more women than men. In addition, we administered metyrapone, which removes glucocorticoid negative feedback, to male and female patients and control subjects in the evening (Young et al. 1994). The response to metyrapone also showed sex differences: depressed women manifested rebound secretion of β-lipotropin and β-endorphin (β-LPH/β-end), which are co-synthesized and released with ACTH (Figure 2–1), in comparison with their matched control subjects (analysis of variance [ANOVA], F = 8.8, $df = 1, P = .01$), while the male patients did not. This result indicates that depressed women, but not depressed men, have increased central HPA drive in the evening.

Table 2–1. Summary of basic and clinical studies of sex differences in hypothalamic-pituitary-adrenal (HPA) axis regulation

Human studies	Findings
	Depressed patients
Young et al. 1991	• Cortisol levels are higher in women than in men.
Young et al. 1994	• β-LPH/β-end response to metyrapone is greater in women than in men.
Young et al. 1993	• Postmenopausal women show more dexamethasone resistance than do premenopausal women.
	Normal subjects
Kirschbaum et al. 1996	• Estrogen increases stress response in men.
Altemus et al. 1997	• Women are less sensitive to dexamethasone feedback during the luteal than during the follicular phase of the menstrual cycle.
Roca et al. 1998a, 1998b	• Progesterone inhibits dexamethasone feedback and increases ACTH response to exercise in leuprolide acetate–treated women.
Young 1995; Young et al. 1991	• Women are less sensitive to cortisol infusion during the luteal phase than during the follicular phase of the menstrual cycle.
Animal studies	
Jones et al. 1972; Young 1996	• Female rats show greater ACTH and cortisol response to stress than do male rats.
Burgess and Handa 1992; Viau and Meaney 1991	• Estrogen inhibits glucocorticoid feedback in ovariectomized female rats.
Keller-Wood et al. 1988	• Progesterone blocks glucocorticoid feedback in ewes.
Vamvakopoulos and Chrousos 1993	• Estrogen increases CRH gene expression in vitro.
Turner and Weaver 1985	• Female rats have a greater number of hippocampal glucocorticoid receptors than do male rats.

Note. ACTH = adrenocorticotropic hormone; β-LPH/β-end = β-lipotropin and β-endorphin; CRH = corticotropin-releasing hormone.

Dexamethasone Nonsuppression, Aging, and Menopause

Sapolsky and colleagues' (1986) glucocorticoid cascade hypothesis suggests that stress and repeated bouts of hypercortisolemia lead to downregulation of glucocorticoid receptors, which in turn results in further glucocorticoid hypersecretion, eventually leading to loss of hippocampal neurons. Sapolsky and associates' studies in rats suggest that aging is a critical variable and that aging rats demonstrate downregulation of glucocorticoid receptors, failure to shut off stress-induced glucocorticoid secretion, and hippocampal neuronal loss. Because aging is also associated with HPA axis dysregulation in depression (Akil et al. 1993; Halbreich et al. 1984; Lewis et al. 1984), our group tested the hypothesis that the repeated episodes of hypercortisolemia that are seen in recurrent depression lead to progressive HPA axis dysregulation.

We conducted these studies in 51 depressed women, 36 of whom were premenopausal and 15 of whom were postmenopausal (Young 1995; Young et al. 1993). This large number of subjects enabled us to examine several factors that might be associated with dexamethasone nonsuppression, including age, recurrent episodes, and menopausal status. We divided patients into those experiencing their first episode of depression versus those with recurrent unipolar depression and examined differences in rates of pituitary nonsuppression. We found no effect of recurrent episodes but observed that, within both recurrent and first-episode subgroups, aging was associated with a higher incidence of HPA axis dysregulation. We also examined possible relationships between the absolute number of depressive episodes, on the one hand, and baseline hormonal measures, postdexamethasone hormonal measures, or suppressor versus nonsuppressor status, on the other. Again, the data did not support the hypothesis that recurrent episodes of depression were associated with progressive HPA axis dysregulation, but rather that aging was the critical variable. Because 16 of the 20 subjects over age 50 years were women, we could not determine whether aging was also a factor in men. However, in women, aging appeared to be a more important factor than the absolute number of episodes.

We were also interested in exploring the role of menopausal status versus age, and the consequent effect of loss of gonadal steroids, on HPA axis regulation in depressed women (Young et al. 1993). We conducted studies using a protocol examining baseline and postdexamethasone secretion of β-LPH/β-end and cortisol over the course of the day (8:00 A.M.–4:00 P.M.). Plasma cortisol concentrations did not differ between menopausal and premenopausal women. However, the premenopausal women demonstrated a significantly lower incidence of pituitary (β-LPH) nonsuppression ($n = 36$; β-LPH/β-end; nonsuppressor = 44%) than did the postmenopausal women ($n = 15$; nonsuppressor = 81%). We used stepwise regression analysis to determine which of a number of potential variables were associated with β-LPH/β-end nonsuppression in women. Independent variables included age, menopausal status, baseline β-LPH/β-end and cortisol, severity of depression as assessed by Hamilton Rating Scale for Depression (Hamilton 1960) scores, and the number of previous episodes of depression. We found that baseline cortisol, menopausal status, and age each had a significant effect on pituitary nonsuppression. However, the best predictor of β-LPH/β-end nonsuppression was menopausal status, which was chosen over age in our regression analysis and, combined with baseline cortisol, yielded a correlation coefficient of .817 (Young 1995).

This suggests that menopausal status, in conjunction with cortisol hypersecretion, is a critical variable in the development of dexamethasone resistance, accounting for 65% of the variance. The fact that pre- and postmenopausal women have similar cortisol levels, whereas premenopausal women are less likely to demonstrate β-LPH/β-end nonsuppression, suggests that gonadal steroids may modulate the HPA axis and exert some protective effect against high levels of endogenous glucocorticoids (cortisol).

In summary, although menopause itself does not appear to be associated with increases in plasma cortisol concentrations in depressed women, it is associated with an increase in dexamethasone resistance in depression. There is a wide variation in cortisol levels in depressed women; however, the ability to suppress dexamethasone is probably a more sensitive marker of the overall integrity of the HPA axis than a single sample of cortisol. Resistance to dexamethasone suppression is strongly associated with increased baseline cortisol secretion and may reflect the development of glucocorticoid receptor downregulation in the hippocampus following a period of hypercortisolemia. The observation that premenopausal women demonstrate normal suppression to dexamethasone suggests that they are more resistant than postmenopausal women to endogenous glucocorticoid–induced glucocorticoid receptor downregulation, perhaps because of the effects of high, or fluctuating, gonadal steroid levels. Increased dexamethasone resistance in postmenopausal women may be indicative of hippocampal dysfunction. Such dysfunction has important clinical implications, because the hippocampus not only is critical for negative feedback regulation of the HPA axis but also plays an important role in memory function, particularly in the acquisition of new information.

These sex differences in HPA axis function are not found exclusively in depressed patients. Studies in animals, and in humans without psychiatric illness, have demonstrated interactions between gonadal steroids and the HPA axis, as well as a sexually dimorphic stress response. These data, which we review in the next section, provide us with an understanding of the basic mechanisms underlying the clinical observation that women have an increased vulnerability to depressive disorders.

Sex Differences in HPA Axis Regulation: Animal Studies

Studies in rodents support the existence of sex differences in several of the elements of the HPA axis. Female rats appear to have a more robust HPA axis response to stress than do male rats, and there is evidence that estrogen is at least partly responsible for this sexual dimorphism. For example, compared with male rats, female rats have a faster onset of corticosterone secretion after stress and a faster rate of rise of corticosterone (Jones et al. 1972). The increased corticosterone response is accompanied by a greatly increased ACTH response to stress in female rodents (Young 1996). Furthermore, corticosteroid-binding globulin (CBG) is positively regulated by estrogen and is thus higher in female rats; however, estrogen and progesterone have been demonstrated to affect the HPA axis independently of the effects of CBG. In addition, chronic estrogen treatment of ovariectomized female rats enhances their corticosterone response to stress and slows their recovery from stress (Burgess and Handa 1992). Studies by Viau and Meaney (1991) demonstrated a greater ACTH and corticosterone stress response in acute estradiol–treated rats compared with ovariectomized female rats or with estradiol-plus-progesterone–treated female rats after short-term (24-hour) but not long-term (48-hour) estradiol treatment. This greater ACTH response in females probably results from a greater central CRH response to stress. Interestingly, a partial estrogen response element is found on the CRH gene that is able to confer estrogen enhancement of CRH expression in CV-1 transfected cells (Vamvakopoulos and Chrousos 1993), thereby providing a mechanism by which estradiol may enhance stress responsiveness in females.

Another mechanism by which estrogen might increase the HPA stress response is through inhibition of glucocorticoid feedback mechanisms. A steeper rate of rise of corticosterone is necessary to elicit glucocorticoid fast feedback in female rats than in male rats (Jones et al. 1972). Two studies (Burgess and Handa 1992; Viau and Meaney 1991) have demonstrated that estrogen treatment delays ACTH and glucocorticoid shutoff following a stress in estrogen-treated female rats compared with ovariectomized female rats. In addition, estradiol treatment blocks downregulation of hippocampal glucocorticoid receptors following chronic administration of RU 28362, a glucocorticoid agonist, in rats. After long-term (21 days) estradiol treatment, the potent and selective glucocorticoid RU 28362 was ineffective in blocking ether-stress-induced ACTH secretion (Burgess and Handa 1992). Although these data may appear to contradict our group's findings that dexamethasone nonsuppression is more common in postmenopausal than in premenopausal women, in all cases estrogen blocks the effect of endogenous glucocorticoids. We postulate that after menopause, an increased sensitivity to glucocorticoids develops and, therefore, that small increases in glucocorticoid secretion during depression lead to greater glucocorticoid receptor downregulation and thus dexamethasone nonsuppression.

There is also evidence to indicate that progesterone, like estrogen, may dampen feedback mechanisms in the HPA axis. Work by Keller-Wood and colleagues (1988) in pregnant ewes and ewes given progesterone infusions has demonstrated that progesterone can diminish the effectiveness of cortisol feedback on stress responsiveness in vivo. In addition, progesterone has antiglucocorticoid effects on feedback in gonadally female rats in vivo and in vitro (Duncan and Duncan 1979; Svec 1988). Progesterone binds to the glucocorticoid receptor; although it binds to the receptor more quickly than does glucocorticoid itself, progesterone binds to a different site on the receptor than do glucocorticoids (Svec 1988). Progesterone can also increase the rate of dissociation of glucocorticoids from the glucocorticoid receptor (Rousseau et al. 1972). In addition, in cultured rat hepatoma cells, dexamethasone and progesterone bind to the same receptor, and progesterone is a clear competitive antagonist of dexamethasone binding. Although the majority of these effects are exerted at the glucocorticoid receptor, binding studies with expressed human mineralocorticoid receptor have demonstrated an affinity of progesterone for the mineralocorticoid receptor in a range similar to that of dexamethasone (Arriza et al. 1987). Furthermore, an increase in mineralocorticoid receptor binding has been seen following progesterone treatment of female rats (Carey et al. 1995). Finally, female rats have a greater number of glucocorticoid receptors in the hippocampus than do male rats (Turner and Weaver 1985), and progesterone modulates glucocorticoid receptor numbers in the hippocampus (Ahima et al. 1992).

Our group designed a series of studies in rats to examine sex differences in sensitivity to glucocorticoid-negative feedback and the extent to which removal of estrogen and progesterone by ovariectomy (an experimental manipulation similar to menopause) affects glucocorticoid negative feedback. Because rats are nocturnal, their pattern of corticosterone secretion is opposite to that of humans; that is, in rats, the morning corresponds to the resting phase and nadir of HPA axis activation, while evening is the active phase and peak of HPA axis activation. We had previously examined two different glucocorticoid administration protocols: corticosterone pellets and corticosterone injections. Both paradigms led to a clear suppression of circadian-driven ACTH and corticosterone secretion, as well as to profound inhibition of the stress response in male rats (Young and Vazquez 1996).

We used these two administration paradigms to block stress responsiveness in the morning and evening in male, intact female, and ovariectomized female rats (Young 1996). In both paradigms, similar responses occurred: 1) failure of exogenous cortisol to block the stress response in intact female rats and 2) increased sensitivity to corticosterone in ovariectomized female rats, making them look more similar to male rats. However, differences remained between the ovariectomized female rats and the male rats, suggesting that not all of the effects of ovarian steroids depend on the presence of ovarian steroid hormones at the time of study (i.e., activational effects), but rather that there may be sex differences dependent upon prenatal effects of steroid hormones on the organization of brain systems (i.e., organizational effects). When we examined the effectiveness of dexamethasone in inhibiting stress responsiveness in male and female rats, we found similar levels of inhibition in male and female rats, suggesting that resistance to corticosterone may involve mechanisms not invoked by dexamethasone, such as mineralocorticoid receptors. The animal literature on sex differences in HPA axis function is summarized in Table 2–1.

Sex Differences in HPA Axis Regulation: Studies in Humans Without Psychiatric Illness

The above data indicate that sexual dimorphism in HPA axis regulation exists in rats and other animals (see Table 2–1). But do similar dimorphisms exist in humans, and, if so, might they contribute to the increased vulnerability of women to depression? Until recently, the lack of a reliable stress test has limited studies on sex differences in stress response. However, with the introduction of the Trier Social Stress Test (Kirschbaum et al. 1995), studies can now be conducted in this area. In the Trier Social Stress Test, subjects undergo a mock job interview in front of a panel of interviewers who are instructed not to provide any verbal or nonverbal feedback. This test is a reliable and robust stressor in normal subjects (Kirschbaum et al. 1995). It has now been shown that oral contraceptives decrease the free cortisol response to a social stressor in women (Kirschbaum et al. 1995), while treatment of normal men with estradiol for 48 hours results in enhanced ACTH and cortisol response to a social stressor (Kirschbaum et al. 1996). These data from studies of estrogen treatment in men are consistent with the results of studies in rats (Burgess and Handa 1992; Viau and Meaney 1991). However, results from studies of oral contraceptives are more difficult to interpret than results from estradiol administration in men, because oral contraceptives are synthetic steroids and may differ from endogenous steroids in their effects.

In addition to investigating HPA axis response to social stress, our group and others have examined sex differences in the response of the HPA axis to pharmacological challenges. For example, we (Young 1995) administered ovine corticotropin-releasing hormone (oCRH) to men and women and found a 40% greater cortisol response in women, again consistent with the findings of animal studies. As oCRH is acting at the level of the pituitary, this suggests differences at the level of the anterior pituitary corticotrope.

In another study, we found that infusion of cortisol "turns off" corticotroph secretion within 15 minutes of the onset of a rise in cortisol in both premenopausal female subjects and age-matched male control subjects (Young 1995; Young et al. 1991). However, after termination of the infusion, men continued to show inhibition of corticotroph secretion for 60 minutes, whereas women began to secrete β-LPH/β-end within this hour. The data indicate that this difference may depend on progesterone. Women with follicular-phase plasma progesterone concentrations (progesterone = 0.26 ± 0.15 ng/mL) exhibited patterns of suppression of β-LPH/β-end secretion similar to those of men. However, women with progesterone concentrations typical of the luteal phase (progesterone = 6.85 ± 0.9 ng/mL) showed rebound β-LPH/β-end secretion following termination of cortisol infusion. Thus, these findings suggest that progesterone antagonizes the feedback effects of cortisol in humans and are thus consistent with the Keller-Wood group's (1988) demonstration of an antagonistic effect of progesterone on the feedback effects of cortisol infusion in ewes. Combined with the in vitro evidence, described earlier, for antagonistic effects of progesterone at the glucocorticoid receptor, these data suggest that progesterone is an important modulator of HPA axis function in humans.

Other human models that can be used to examine the interactions between gonadal steroids and the HPA axis are pregnancy and the menstrual cycle, since both involve fluctuations in gonadal steroid levels. In pregnancy, increases in both estrogen and progesterone occur. Increases in plasma CBG and cortisol during pregnancy are also well documented, and dexamethasone challenge studies indicate resistance to glucocorticoid negative feedback during pregnancy (Carr et al. 1981; Demey-Ponsart et al. 1982; Nolten and Rueckert 1981). However, the degree to which postdexamethasone hypercortisolism is simply an artifact of increased CBG levels, leading to higher levels of plasma cortisol following dexamethasone administration, is not completely known. Although dexamethasone itself is not bound by CBG, pregnancy could alter the metabolism of dexamethasone, resulting in less dexamethasone bioavailability. At least one study (Nolten and Rueckert 1981) has demonstrated higher free cortisol during pregnancy, higher free cortisol production following an ACTH infusion, decreased suppression of free cortisol by dexamethasone, and a normal circadian rhythm of cortisol, pointing to a change in cortisol set point during pregnancy. Again, these data are compatible with those showing that both estrogen and progesterone can antagonize the effects of glucocorticoids on negative feedback.

With respect to the menstrual cycle, recent studies by Altemus and colleagues (1997) have found increased resistance to dexamethasone suppression during the luteal phase of the menstrual cycle as compared with the follicular phase, a change that may again be related to either increased estradiol or increased progesterone during the luteal phase. Furthermore, ovarian steroids influenced the expression of glucocorticoid receptor mRNA in lymphocytes, resulting in a decrease in glucocorticoid receptors in the luteal phase compared with the follicular phase of the menstrual cycle (Altemus et al. 1997) and suggesting that decreases in glucocorticoid receptors may explain the decreased response to dexamethasone. Using a design that allowed them to distinguish the effects of progesterone from those of estrogen, Roca and co-workers (1998a, 1998b) studied normal women first treated with leuprolide acetate, a gonadotropin-releasing hormone (GnRH) agonist that causes suppression of both estrogen and progesterone secretion, and then given sequential replacement of estrogen and progesterone. Roca and colleagues examined the subjects' response to exercise stress as well as to dexamethasone feedback and found that the exercise stress response was increased and the response to dexamethasone feedback was decreased during the progesterone "add-back" phase but not during the estrogen add-back phase. Again, these data suggest that progesterone acts as a glucocorticoid antagonist. Thus, so far, the data from human studies suggest that ovarian steroids, particularly progesterone, influence the HPA axis response to stress by modulating sensitivity to negative feedback. Furthermore, some data suggest that progesterone may have negative effects on mood, particularly in women with premenstrual dysphoric disorder (PMDD), in which depressive symptoms occur during the luteal phase of the menstrual cycle, when progesterone levels are high. Although the exact role of sex hormones in PMDD has not been established (Hammarback et al. 1985), estrogen and progesterone suppression with leuprolide acetate has been reported to produce significant symptom improvement in depression (Rosenbaum et al. 1996) and PMDD (Mortola et al. 1991).

Discussion

In this review we have examined the interactions between gonadal steroids and the HPA axis, and the ability of gonadal steroids to modulate glucocorticoid negative feedback. We have focused our review and our experimental work on females, and in particular on comparisons between women with and without low levels of gonadal steroids and between premenopausal and postmenopausal women. Although it is possible that gonadal steroids may also modulate HPA axis activity in males, we have chosen to focus on females and the removal of ovarian steroids because 1) our previous studies in depressed women, summarized earlier in this chapter, suggest that ovarian steroids are an important modulator of HPA axis activity in depressed women, producing differences between premenopausal and postmenopausal depressed women; 2) the actions of estrogen and progesterone on HPA axis activity have been well documented in the literature; and 3) whereas testosterone levels in men are relatively stable over months and years well into old age, women undergo monthly cyclical changes in which estrogen effects dominate during the early follicular phase and progesterone effects, in conjunction with estrogen, are prominent during the luteal phase. In addition, loss of ovarian steroids (i.e., menopause) occurs naturally in women, whereas a parallel condition does not occur in men. Therefore, the effects of testosterone loss on the HPA axis of males have less general physiological relevance for understanding the effects of HPA axis function in humans.

From the studies reviewed here, it is clear that ovarian steroids play a modulatory role in HPA axis regulation. However, which of the ovarian steroids is critical is not yet completely clear, given that both estrogen and progesterone appear to have effects. Nor is it clear at which level of the HPA axis the gonadal steroids act. Although substantial experimental evidence supports an antiglucocorticoid effect of progesterone in sheep and humans, and studies demonstrate a modulatory site for progesterone on glucocorticoid receptors, it is also likely that estrogen plays a role in females' increased resistance to HPA feedback inhibition. Studies in both rodents and humans (Kirschbaum et al. 1996; Viau and Meaney 1991; Young et al. 1995) have demonstrated that estrogen treatment enhances stress responsiveness. Estrogen may inhibit glucocorticoid feedback mechanisms by altering glucocorticoid receptors (Burgess and Handa 1992) or by increasing CRH mRNA levels and thus increasing CRH anterior pituitary peptide stores (Vamvakopoulos and Chrousos 1993). However, it is unlikely that sex differences in resistance to glucocorticoid suppression can be accounted for by sex differences in the number of glucocorticoid receptors (Turner and Weaver 1985), since females have higher numbers of receptors than males.

The finding of an increased ACTH response to stress in ovariectomized female rats compared with male rats has important implications for our understanding of stress and stress responsiveness in women. Several stress-associated disorders are more common in women—for example, depression and anxiety disorders, including posttraumatic stress disorder (PTSD) (Breslau et al. 1991; Kessler et al. 1994). If indeed there is an exaggerated central CRH response to stress in women, this may partially explain women's increased susceptibility to these disorders. Additionally, resistance to the feedback effects of endogenous glucocorticoids, as previously described, may contribute to the increased incidence of stress-related conditions in women. Indeed, Munck and Guyre (1986) have hypothesized that the purpose of glucocorticoids is to terminate not just the HPA axis stress response but the entire stress response. For example, recent studies have suggested that glucocorticoids can inhibit the autonomic nervous system response (McEwen 1995), a finding that supports a role for glucocorticoids in terminating stress-induced activation of the autonomic stress system. Thus, women's increased resistance to glucocorticoids in comparison with men could exaggerate stress responsiveness in a number of physiological systems.

In summary, as described earlier in this chapter, it is possible that gonadal steroid antagonism of glucocorticoid feedback mechanisms, and the increased stress responsiveness of females, contributes to the increased prevalence of anxiety disorders and autonomic hyperarousal in women compared with men. In addition, as previously noted, organizational differences between male and female brains are caused by exposure to high levels of gonadal steroids in the pre- and perinatal periods. The interactions of these organizational effects in females with cyclical gonadal steroid hormone changes after puberty, followed then by menopause and the loss of these same steroids, suggest that stress responsiveness and susceptibility to stress-related disorders could vary substantially over women's lifetimes. There is certainly evidence that women's increased vulnerability to depression arises at puberty, a time when gonadal steroids can further enhance stress responsiveness (Kessler et al. 1993). Additionally, the evidence linking stress and glucocorticoids to hippocampal damage and subsequent memory problems (Issa et al. 1990), and the important role that gonadal steroids may play in protection from these effects in premenopausal women, implies that further research is needed into the interaction of stress, menopause, and memory impairment.

References

Ahima RS, Lawson ANL, Osei SYS, et al: Sexual dimorphism in regulation of type II corticosteroid receptor immunoreactivity in the rat hippocampus. Endocrinology 131:1409–1416, 1992

Akil H, Haskett R, Young EA, et al: Multiple HPA profiles in endogenous depression: effect of age and sex on cortisol and beta-endorphin. Biol Psychiatry 33:73–85, 1993

Altemus M, Redwine L, Yung-Mei L, et al: Reduced sensitivity to glucocorticoid feedback and reduced glucocorticoid receptor mRNA expression in the luteal phase of the menstrual cycle. Neuropsychopharmacology 17:100–109, 1997

Arriza JL, Weinberger C, Cerelli G, et al: Cloning of human mineralocorticoid receptor complementary DNA: structural and functional kinship with the glucocorticoid receptor. Science 237:268–275, 1987

Birnberg NC, Civelli O, Lissitzski JC, et al: Regulation of pro-opiomelanocortin gene expression in the pituitary and central nervous system. Endocrinology 110:134A, 1982

Birnberg NC, Lissitzky JC, Hinman M, et al: Glucocorticoids regulate proopiomelanocortin gene expression in vivo at the levels of transcription and secretion. Proc Natl Acad Sci U S A 80:6982–6986, 1983

Breslau N, Davis GC, Andreski P, et al: Traumatic events and posttraumatic stress disorder in an urban population of young adults. Arch Gen Psychiatry 48:216–222, 1991

Brown GW, Harris T: Social Origins of Depression: A Study of Psychiatric Disorder in Women. New York, Free Press, 1978

Burgess LH, Handa RJ: Chronic estrogen-induced alterations in adrenocorticotropin and corticosterone secretion, and glucocorticoid receptor-mediated functions in female rats. Endocrinology 131: 1261–1269, 1992

Carey MP, Deterd CH, de Koning J, et al: The influence of ovarian steroids on hypothalamic-pituitary-adrenal regulation in the female rat. J Endocrinol 144:311–332, 1995

Carr BR, Parker CR Jr, Madden JD, et al: Maternal plasma adrenocorticotropin and cortisol relationships throughout human pregnancy. Am J Obstet Gynecol 139:416–422, 1981

Carroll BJ, Curtis GC, Mendels J: Neuroendocrine regulation in depression, I: limbic system-adrenocortical dysfunction. Arch Gen Psychiatry 33:1039–1044, 1976

Childs GV, Morell JL, Niendorf A, et al: Cytochemical studies of corticotropin releasing factor (CRF) receptors in anterior lobe corticotrophs: binding, glucocorticoid regulation and endocytosis of [Biotinyl-Ser1] CRF. Endocrinology 119:2129–2142, 1986

de Kloet R, Wallach G, McEwen BS: Differences in corticosterone and dexamethasone binding to rat brain and pituitary. Endocrinology 96:598–609, 1975

Demey-Ponsart E, Foidart JM, Sulon J, et al: Serum CBG, free and total cortisol and circadian patterns of adrenal function in normal pregnancy. Journal of Steroid Biochemistry 16:165–169, 1982

Duncan MR, Duncan GR: An in vivo study of the action of antiglucocorticoids on thymus weight ratio, antibody titre and the adrenal-pituitary-hypothalamus axis. Journal of Steroid Biochemistry 10: 245–259, 1979

Frank E, Anderson B, Reynolds C, et al: Life events and the research diagnostic criteria endogenous subtype: a confirmation of the distinction using the Bedford College methods. Arch Gen Psychiatry 51: 519–524, 1994

Halbreich U, Asnis GM, Zumoff B, et al: The effect of age and sex on cortisol secretion depressives and normals. Psychiatry Res 13:221–229, 1984

Hamilton M: A rating scale for depression. J Neurol Neurosurg Psychiatry 23:56–62, 1960

Hammarback S, Backstrom T, Holst J, et al: Cyclical mood changes as in the premenstrual tension syndrome during sequential estrogen-progestogen postmenopausal replacement therapy. Acta Obstet Gynecol Scand 64:393–397, 1985

Herman JP, Schafer MK-H, Young EA, et al: Hippocampal regulation of the hypothalamo-pituitary-adrenocortical axis: in situ hybridization analysis of CRF and vasopressin messenger RNA expression in the hypothalamic paraventricular nucleus following hippocampectomy. J Neurosci 9:3072–3082, 1989

Issa AM, Rowe W, Meaney MJ: Hypothalamic-pituitary-adrenal activity in aged, cognitively impaired and cognitively unimpaired rats. J Neurosci 10:3247–3254, 1990

Jones MT, Brush FR, Neame RLB: Characteristics of fast feedback control of corticotrophin release by corticosteroids. J Endocrinol 55:489–497, 1972

Keller-Wood M, Silbiger J, Wood CE: Progesterone attenuates the inhibition of adrenocorticotropin responses by cortisol in nonpregnant ewes. Endocrinology 123:647–651, 1988

Kendler KS, Kessler RC, Walters EE, et al: Stressful life events, genetic liability, and onset of an episode of major depression in women. Am J Psychiatry 152:833–842, 1995

Kessler RC, McGonagle KA, Swartz M, et al: Sex and depression in the National Comorbidity Survey, I: lifetime prevalence, chronicity and recurrence. J Affect Disord 29:85–96, 1993

Kessler RC, McGonagle KA, Zhao S, et al: Lifetime and 12-month prevalence of DSM-III-R psychiatric disorders in the United States. Arch Gen Psychiatry 51:8–19, 1994

Kirschbaum C, Pirke K-M, Hellhammer DH: Preliminary evidence for reduced cortisol responsivity to psychological stress in women using oral contraceptive medication. Psychoneuroendocrinology 20:509–514, 1995

Kirschbaum C, Schommer N, Federenko I, et al: Short-term estradiol treatment enhances pituitary-adrenal axis and sympathetic responses to psychosocial stress in healthy young men. J Clin Endocrinol Metab 81:3639–3643, 1996

Lewis DA, Pfohl B, Schlecte J, et al: Influence of age on the cortisol response to dexamethasone. Psychiatry Res 13:213–220, 1984

McEwen B: Adrenal steroid actions on brain dissecting the fine line between protection and damage, in Neurobiological and Clinical Consequences of Stress: From Normal Adaptation to PTSD. Edited by Friedman MJ, Charney DS, Deutch AY. Philadelphia, PA, Lippincott-Raven, 1995, pp 135–147

McEwen BS, Weiss JM, Schwartz LS: Selective retention of corticosterone by limbic structures in the rat brain. Nature 220:911–913, 1968

McEwen BS, Weiss JM, Schwartz LS: Retention of corticosterone by cell nuclei from brain regions of adrenalectomized rats. Brain Res 17:471–482, 1970

Mortola JF, Girton L, Fischer U: Successful treatment of severe premenstrual syndrome by combined use of gonadotropin-releasing hormone agonist and estrogen/progestin. J Clin Endocrinol Metab 72:252A–252F, 1991

Munck A, Guyre PM: Glucocorticoid physiology, pharmacology and stress. Adv Exp Med Biol 196:81–96, 1986

Nolten WE, Rueckert PA: Elevated free cortisol index in pregnancy: possible regulatory mechanisms. Am J Obstet Gynecol 139:492–498, 1981

Reul JMH, de Kloet ER: Two receptor systems for corticosterone in rat brain: microdistribution and differential occupation. Endocrinology 117:2505–2511, 1985

Roberts JL, Budarf ML, Baxter JD, et al: Selective reduction of pro-adrenocorticotropin/andorphin proteins and messenger ribonucleic acid activity in mouse pituitary tumor cells by glucocorticoids. Biochemistry 18:4907–4915, 1979

Roca AC, Altemus M, Galliven E, et al: Effect of reproductive hormones on the hypothalamic-pituitary-adrenal axis response to stress (abstract). Biol Psychiatry 43:6S, 1998a

Roca CA, Schmidt PJ, Altemus M, et al: Effects of reproductive steroids on the hypothalamic-pituitary-adrenal axis response to low dose dexamethasone. Abstract of paper presented at Neuroendocrine Workshop on Stress, New Orleans, LA, June 21–23, 1998b

Rosenbaum AH, Ginsburg K, Rosenberg R, et al: Treatment of major depression and manic-depressive illness with gonadotropin-releasing hormone-agonist therapy. Abstract of paper presented at International Society of Psychoneuroendocrinology XXVIIth Congress, Cascais, Portugal, August 1996

Rousseau GG, Baxter JD, Tomkins GM: Glucocorticoid receptors: relations between steroid binding and biological effects. J Mol Biol 67:99–115, 1972

Sachar EJ, Hellman L, Roffwarg HP, et al: Disrupted 24-hour patterns of cortisol secretion in psychotic depressives. Arch Gen Psychiatry 28:19–24, 1973

Sapolsky RM, Krey LC, McEwen BS: The neuroendocrinology of stress and aging: the glucocorticoid cascade hypothesis. Endocr Rev 7:284–301, 1986

Schachter BS, Johnson LK, Baxter JD, et al: Differential regulation by glucocorticoids of proopiomelanocortin mRNA levels in the anterior and intermediate lobes of the rat pituitary. Endocrinology 110:1142–1444, 1982

Schwartz J, Billestrup N, Perrin M, et al: Identification of cortico-tropin-releasing factor (CRF) target cells and effects of dexamethasone on binding in anterior pituitary using a fluorescent analog of CRF. Endocrinology 119:2376–2382, 1986

Svec F: Differences in the interaction of RU 486 and ketoconazole with the second binding site of the glucocorticoid receptor. Endocrinology 123:1902–1906, 1988

Turner BB, Weaver DA: Sexual dimorphism of glucocorticoid binding in rat brain. Brain Res 343:16–23, 1985

Vamvakopoulos NC, Chrousos GP: Evidence of direct estrogenic regulation of human corticotropin-releasing hormone gene expression: potential implications for the sexual dimorphism of the stress response and immune/inflammatory reaction. J Clin Invest 92:1896–1902, 1993

Viau V, Meaney MJ: Variations in the hypothalamic-pituitary-adrenal response to stress during the estrous cycle in the rat. Endocrinology 129:2503–2511, 1991

Young EA: Glucocorticoid cascade hypothesis revisited: role of gonadal steroids. Depression 3:20–27, 1995

Young EA: Sex differences in response to exogenous corticosterone. Mol Psychiatry 1:313–319, 1996

Young EA, Vazquez D: Hypercortisolemia, hippocampal glucocorticoid receptors, and fast feedback. Mol Psychiatry 1:149–159, 1996

Young EA, Haskett RF, Watson SJ, et al: Loss of glucocorticoid fast feedback in depression. Arch Gen Psychiatry 48:693–699, 1991

Young EA, Kotun J, Haskett RF, et al: Dissociation between pituitary and adrenal suppression to dexamethasone in depression. Arch Gen Psychiatry 50:395–403, 1993

Young EA, Haskett RF, Grunhaus L, et al: Increased evening activation of the hypothalamic pituitary adrenal axis in depressed patients. Arch Gen Psychiatry 51:701–707, 1994

Young EA, Kwak SP, Kottak J: Negative feedback regulation following administration of chronic exogenous corticosterone. J Neuroendocrinol 7:37

Chapter 3

Modulation of Anxiety by Reproductive Hormones

Margaret Altemus, M.D., and
Elizabeth Kagan Arleo, B.A.

As detailed throughout this volume, multiple clinical observations indicate that gender and reproductive hormones have a major impact on the prevalence and course of mood and anxiety disorders. Identification of the physiological processes underlying these sex differences and the effects of reproductive hormone fluctuations on mood and anxiety disorders should provide a better understanding of the pathophysiology of depression and anxiety and should potentially suggest new treatment approaches.

Recent work has begun to show that gonadal steroids and sex are important modulators of both hormonal stress response systems (see Chapter 2, this volume) and behavioral responses to stress, including anxiety. In this chapter we will first review the cellular mechanism of action of behaviorally active reproductive hormones and present a brief overview of stress response physiology, then focus on the effects of gender and reproductive hormones on anxiety in humans and in animal models of anxiety. We will also review the effects of gender and gonadal steroids on some potentially relevant aspects of brain neurochemistry, structure, and function that are not covered in other chapters in this volume.

Cellular Mechanisms of Reproductive Hormone Action

Familial data indicate that the increased vulnerability of women to affective disorders is not an X-linked trait (Merikangas et al.

1985). Instead, increased vulnerability in women appears to arise from interactions of sex-specific hormonal and environmental factors with non-sex-specific genes on other chromosomes. Fluctuations in reproductive hormone levels occur in both sexes in utero and in women during puberty, the menstrual cycle, pregnancy, lactation, and menopause. Although reproductive hormone levels in men are comparatively stable, there is a rise in androgens at puberty and a gradual reduction in androgen production with age. Reproductive hormones that have been examined for their effects on anxiety and anxiety-associated neural systems include the gonadal steroids (estrogen, progesterone, and androgens) and oxytocin, a neuropeptide secreted during lactation. It is important to keep in mind that sex differences in mood and anxiety can arise both from the acute effects of fluctuations in reproductive hormones and from sexual differentiation of brain structure and function during development (McEwen et al. 1997). Gonadal steroids can affect brain systems known to mediate mood and anxiety on multiple levels, through alterations in neural structure, neurotransmitter and neuropeptide signaling efficiency, neuronal excitability, and synaptic plasticity.

Intracellular gonadal steroid receptors have been identified in multiple brain areas previously implicated in the regulation of mood and autonomic reactivity, including the hypothalamus, the amygdala, the hippocampus, the bed nucleus of the stria terminalis, and the locus coeruleus (Simerly et al. 1990). Gonadal steroids easily pass into neurons and bind to intracellular receptors. Once hormone is bound, the receptor is "activated" and can then move into the nucleus to act as a transcription factor to regulate gene expression. The effects of circulating steroid hormones can be controlled in particular brain areas by the presence or absence of various steroid receptor subtypes and receptor isoforms, each having a different activity (Auricchio 1989; Kuiper et al. 1997), and by transcriptional co-factors, which can modify the effects of the activated receptor on gene transcription (Katzenellenbogen et al. 1996). An additional level of complexity was added with the discovery that after estrogen is bound, estrogen receptors can alter the activity of other steroid hormone transcription factors, including activated glucocorticoid, thyroid, and progesterone receptors (Meyer et al. 1989; Uht et al. 1997; Zhu et al. 1996). In addition, induction of androgen-metabolizing enzyme activity in specific brain areas regulates the activity of androgen hormones. Testosterone can be locally metabolized to dihydrotestosterone, a hormone with relatively high affinity for the androgen receptor, or to androstenedione, a hormone with lower affinity for the androgen receptor, or can be metabolized by aromatase to estradiol, causing activation of estrogen, rather than androgen, receptors. Males and females have similar densities of estrogen receptors in extrahypothalamic brain areas relevant to anxiety, including the hippocampus, the raphe nucleus, and the cortex.

In addition to affecting gene transcription through binding to the classical intracellular steroid receptors as described above, gonadal steroids appear to have the capability to act directly at neuronal membranes. These direct membrane actions of gonadal steroids occur within seconds or minutes, which is much more rapid than the time required for gene transcription and protein synthesis through the intracellular receptor. Direct membrane actions of gonadal steroids appear to include uncoupling of intracellular G protein–coupled second-messenger systems, regulation of ion channels, modification of neurotransmitter receptor structure, and ultrastructural membrane remodeling (Wong et al. 1996).

Several steroid hormone metabolites are classified as "neurosteroids" because they can be synthesized by neurons and glial cells in the central nervous system (CNS) (Robel and Baulieu 1995). Many of the neurosteroid hormones are produced both locally in the brain and outside the brain by the gonads and adrenal glands, from which neurosteroid hormones enter the circulation and then pass into the brain. Thus, the action of these neurosteroid hormones can be tied to fluctuations in peripheral hormone and hormone precursor levels that occur during pregnancy, across the menstrual cycle, and during stress. Neurosteroids seem to modulate neurotransmission primarily by acting directly on the neuronal membrane, but also may have direct effects on gene transcription (Rupprecht et al. 1996). Neurosteroids have been shown to modulate dopamine release from

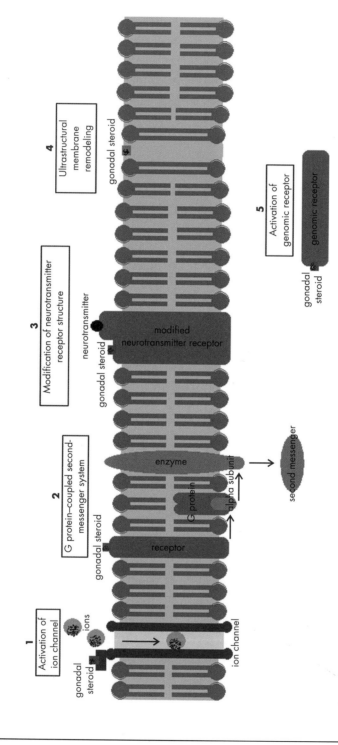

Figure 3–1. Proposed mechanisms of gonadal steroid action: 1) activation of ion channel, 2) G protein–coupled second-messenger system, 3) modification of neurotransmitter receptor structure, 4) ultrastructural membrane remodeling, and 5) activation of genomic receptor.

striatal neurons, and modulate functioning of gamma-aminobutyric acid type A (GABA$_A$) receptors, glutamatergic N-methyl-D-aspartic acid (NMDA) receptors, and the nicotinic acetylcholine receptor. Some neurosteroids have excitatory and others have inhibitory effects on neuronal activity and behavior. One of the most well-studied effects of neurosteroids is the potent facilitation of GABA action at GABA$_A$ receptors by pregnenolone sulfate and allopregnanolone, two progesterone metabolites. These steroids have anesthetic, hypnotic, and anxiolytic effects and mimic the effects of benzodiazepines, which act at an adjacent site within the GABA$_A$ receptor complex.

Another reproductive hormone likely to modulate anxiety and stress responses is the neuropeptide oxytocin. Oxytocin is synthesized in the hypothalamus and secreted both into the brain and into the circulation. Oxytocin stimulates smooth-muscle contractions in several parts of the body. Oxytocin stimulates penile contractions during sexual activity, stimulates uterine contractions during labor, and stimulates expulsion of milk during lactation. In the brain, oxytocin directs coordinated behavioral effects, including facilitation of mating and parental behaviors and enhancement of analgesia, and also seems to play a role in satiety signaling after eating, drinking, and sexual activity (McCarthy and Altemus 1997). Oxytocin, like other neuropeptides, appears to act exclusively at membrane receptors, which in turn activate intracellular second-messenger systems.

Relationship of Stress Physiology to Anxiety

Anxiety is a state of cognitive and autonomic hyperarousal that is adaptive in stressful situations, producing enhanced vigilance, learning, and reactivity. Yet in some individuals, anxiety reaches a level that is counterproductive or even incapacitating. Anxiety responses to stress are self-limited in healthy individuals but exaggerated and prolonged in patients with anxiety disorders. Anxiety disorders, including panic disorder, social phobia, obsessive-compulsive disorder (OCD), and posttraumatic stress disorder (PTSD), can be conceptualized as exaggerated fearfulness and a failure to adequately counterregulate the stress response. Depression also can be conceptualized as a more enduring or pervasive reaction to prolonged stress, with a similar loss of the normal homeostatic regulation of the stress response, but also including prominent features of hypothalamic-pituitary-adrenal (HPA) axis hyperactivity, fatigue, anhedonia, and hopelessness (Gold et al. 1988). Consistent with this model is the extremely high comorbidity of depression and anxiety disorders and the high association of depression and anxiety disorders within families (Kendler 1996).

Progress in understanding the neurobiology of stress has provided critical insights into the pathophysiology of anxiety and depression. Recent work has begun to show that gonadal steroids and sex are important modulators of hormonal stress response systems (see Chapter 2, this volume) and behavioral responses to stress. Although a wide variety of neurotransmitters and neuromodulators are activated in response to stress, corticotropin-releasing hormone (CRH), vasopressin, and norepinephrine are considered the principal effectors of the stress response (Chrousos and Gold 1992). The assumption that anxiety disorder and depression pathophysiology involves exaggerated responses to stress is supported by evidence that brain CRH, vasopressin, and noradrenergic systems are hyperactivated in patients with these disorders (Altemus et al. 1992; Charney et al. 1987; Bremner et al. 1997). These systems are also hyperactivated in animal models of anxiety disorders (Coplan et al. 1996; Heim et al. 1997). In addition, in animals, intracerebral administration of mediators of the stress response, particularly CRH, vasopressin, and catecholamines, produces symptoms characteristic of human anxiety disorders, including tachycardia, increased blood pressure, shortness of breath, hypervigilance, reduced sleep, reduced appetite, reduced sexual activity, and increased startle response. Pharmacological challenge studies have linked excess noradrenergic activity to both panic attacks (Charney et al. 1987) and PTSD (Southwick et al. 1993). Moreover, chronic antidepressant treatment, which is clearly effective for treatment of both anxiety disorders and depression in humans, restrains stress response systems at multiple sites by reducing CRH and tyrosine hydroxylase activity, enhancing glucocorticoid receptor activity (Brady et al. 1991), and downregulating arousal-producing β-adrenergic receptors (Heninger and Charney 1987). Chronic treatment with antidepressant agents also reduces behavioral and endocrine responses to stress (Murua and Molina 1992; Reul et al. 1993). Furthermore, benzodiazepines, another clearly effective treatment for anxiety disorders and acute fear, also restrain stress responsivity, as measured by adrenocorticotropin, corticosterone, and catecholamine responses to stress (Breier et al. 1992). Another line of evidence linking stress to the generation of anxiety and depression is the finding that chronic stress and glucocorticoids exaggerate development of fear behaviors in animals (Corodimas et al. 1994; Roozendaal and McGaugh 1996).

Serotonergic systems also play an important role in both stress responsivity and anxiety. A leading hypothesis in the field, primarily based on animal studies and on the anxiolytic efficacy of serotonin reuptake blockers, postulates that some forms of anxiety disorders may be the result of a relative deficiency of serotonin. Preclinical studies indicate that chronic administration of serotonin reuptake blockers increases the efficiency of serotonergic neurotransmission in rats (elMansari et al. 1995). To date, 14 serotonin (5-hydroxytryptamine [5-HT]) receptor subtypes have been identified, some of which may have separate and opposing actions with reference to anxiety. For example, activation of the 5-HT_3 postsynaptic receptor seems to produce anxiogenic effects, while activation of the 5-HT_{1A} and possibly the 5-HT_{2C} postsynaptic receptors seems to have a more anxiolytic effect.

Animal Models of Anxiety

Animal models are a crucial bridge between basic neuroscience and clinical psychiatric research. Clearly, limited methods exist for assessing gender differences and reproductive-related changes in brain neurochemistry, structure, and function in human subjects. Direct measurements of brain neurochemistry and function cannot be made safely in humans, and fresh postmortem tissue from nonmedicated subjects is rarely available. Also, because no specific receptor antagonists are available for human use and because of the side effects associated with manipulation of gonadal steroids, it is difficult to pharmacologically modify reproductive hormones in humans. As a result of these difficulties, few controlled studies to date have examined the effects of reproductive hormones on anxiety disorders in humans.

However, both animal behavioral models of anxiety and direct studies of the effects of gonadal steroids and other reproductive hormones on brain function in animals can be used to identify biochemical mechanisms that may contribute to sex differences in the prevalence and course of anxiety disorders. Animal models also provide an opportunity to manipulate single environmental variables and to control other variables to a degree that would not be possible in human subjects. Unfortunately, to date, most research in animal models of anxiety has involved only male rats or primates—or if both sexes have been used, studies have not examined potential sex differences. This lack of attention to sex differences in animal studies parallels the lack of attention to gender differences in clinical psychiatric research.

A major shortcoming of working with animal models is that there is no access to subjective experience. In humans, anxiety is primarily a subjective state, although it is often accompanied by observable behaviors and physical signs. Also, because the neocortex is much less developed in rodents compared with humans or even primates, it is probably unreasonable to expect parallel subjective experiences of mood to occur in rodent models of psychiatric illness. However, a number of observable behaviors in animals—for example, reduced social interaction, reduced exploratory behavior, and potentiated startle response—mirror anxiety-associated behaviors in humans.

Another difficulty in extrapolating from animal models to humans is that complex social conditions that may contribute to the development of mood and anxiety disorders in humans, such as sexual trauma and economic disadvantages, cannot be reproduced in animals in laboratory environments. However, animal models of anxiety and depression induced by acute social stress are being actively investigated (Albeck et al. 1997). Traumatic and nurturant rearing conditions also have been shown to influence adult anxiety-associated behaviors and brain neurochemistry (Coplan et al. 1996; Heim et al. 1997; Liu et al. 1997).

Another important caveat to keep in mind is that because psychiatric disorders may occur most often in individuals with particular genetic or physiological vulnerabilities, some disorders may be best modeled by particular animal species or particular strains within those species that have biological vulnerabilities similar to those of affected humans. Some strains of rats and some genetically related groups of primates (Suomi 1991) have been shown to be physiologically prone to developing anxiety responses. Examples include the Maudsley Reactive and Roman Low-Avoidance rat strains and the Fawn-Hooded rat strain (Altemus 1995), which has impaired neuronal storage of serotonin. As in humans, where the evidence points to normal hormone levels but exaggerated brain reactivity to the hormones in women with reproductive-related mood disorders (Rubinow et al. 1988; Schmidt et al. 1998), some strains of animals are more sensitive than others to the effects of gonadal steroids (Prasad et al. 1997; Steimer et al. 1997).

A final difficulty in the application of animal models to human illnesses is interspecies differences—that is, the possibility that the biological mechanisms that determine behavior in animals may not function similarly in humans. However, despite the fact that animal models are clearly not identical to human anxiety states or depression, and that the human neocortex is much more complex than the rat neocortex, analogies between animal models and the human state of anxiety are often surprisingly strong, both physiologically and behaviorally. It is not necessary that an animal model match a human disorder in all aspects—phenomenology (face validity), etiology and pathophysiology (construct validity), and drug response (predictive validity)—for the model to be useful in advancing our understanding of the pathophysiology of anxiety (Henn and McKinney 1987; Willner 1991).

A wide range of behavioral models have been developed that mimic the phenomenology of anxiety disorders. Among the most valuable and intensely studied paradigms have been stress-induced models of depression and anxiety. Animal models of anxiety involve induction of fear behavior or distress, with or without classical conditioning of the fear. Conditioned fear paradigms are thought to closely model panic disorder and PTSD, whereas unconditioned fear paradigms are believed to be similar to generalized anxiety disorder. Models of unconditioned fear include separation in young animals, exposure to novel environments, and exposure to noxious stimuli. Behavioral measures of fear or anxiety in these models include freezing (immobility), avoidance behavior, distress cries, and attempts to hide or bury sources of aversive stimuli. One of the most widely used animal models of depression is the learned helplessness—or behavioral despair—model, in which impaired learning and escape behaviors, decreased food intake, and decreased activity occur as a result of exposure to uncontrollable stresses (Maier and Seligman 1976). Behaviors characteristic of the learned helplessness syndrome are reduced by a variety of drugs that act as antidepressants in humans. Although the learned helplessness paradigm is best known as an animal model of depression, it has an equally good phenomenological and therapeutic correspondence to human anxiety syndromes (Drugan et al. 1985).

Models of conditioned fear involve pairing an aversive stimulus with a neutral stimulus and then using the neutral stimulus to induce "fear" behavior or anxiety. Commonly used conditioned-fear models entail presentation of an environmental cue previously paired with footshock (conditioned freezing), presentation of a shock-associated environmental cue coincident with a loud noise (fear-potentiated startle), and performance of a learned behavior that allows escape from shock (conditioned avoidance). Another commonly used paradigm for animal models of anxiety pairs rewards for which the animal must perform some behavior (e.g., lever pressing for food or water) with an aversive stimulus (e.g., an electric shock), producing a "conflict." Rats are motivated to press the lever for food but know that they will receive a shock as well. Agents are defined as anxiolytic if they produce an increased rate of responses punished by the shock (i.e., punished responding), whereas anxiogenic agents have the opposite effect. The assumption in this model is that anxiety produces an exaggerated estimate of the intensity of aversive stimuli.

Gender and Reproductive
Hormone Effects on Anxiety

Estrogen

Several lines of evidence suggest that estrogen has anxiolytic effects. First, multiple studies in rats have shown that estrogen administration to ovariectomized rats reduces conditioned active avoidance behavior (Diaz-Veliz et al. 1991). Estrogen also appears to increase exploration in an open field (A. Gray and Levine 1964; McCarthy 1995) and in the open, exposed arms of the elevated plus-maze (Farr et al. 1995; Nomikos and Spiraki 1988). In addition, estrogen appears to reduce immobility reactions to stimuli previously associated with footshock (fear conditioning) (Altemus et al. 1998). Estrogen also accelerates extinction of passive avoidance behavior (Rivas-Arancibia and Vazquez-Pereyra 1994). Finally, estrogen enhances the anxiolytic effects of several compounds, including intracerebrally administered diazepam and intraventricularly administered oxytocin (McCarthy 1995). These biochemical observations have behavioral correlates, in that estrogen has been shown to enhance the anxiolytic, maternal, and sexual effects of oxytocin in animals. The anxiolytic effect of estrogen seems to be a genomic rather than a rapid membrane effect, since peak effects are seen 48 hours after estrogen administration (Diaz-Veliz et al. 1989).

A few clinical studies have yielded findings consistent with these data, suggesting that estrogen can blunt anxiety. Subclinical anxiety symptoms are reduced in postmenopausal women receiving estrogen replacement therapy (Ditkoff et al. 1991; Wiklund et al. 1993), and estrogen appears to blunt autonomic (heart rate and blood pressure) responses to stress in postmenopausal women (Lindheim et al. 1992). There have been no clinical studies of the effects of estrogen treatment in patients with clinically diagnosed anxiety disorders.

Estrogen-induced reduction in anxiety or fear may not be independent of estrogen's effects on memory. In studies of male and female rats, estrogen appears to enhance memory through actions in the hippocampus (Dohanich et al. 1994; Luine 1994; Packard and Teather 1997; Singh et al. 1994). Human studies also indicate that estrogen can enhance verbal recall in healthy women (Kampen and Sherwin 1994), reduce the incidence of Alzheimer's disease in women (Paganini-Hill and Henderson 1994), and improve memory in women with Alzheimer's disease (Ohkura et al. 1995). Although "memory" should enhance the salience of an aversive event such as footshock conditioning, it may also increase the salience of subsequent experiences in which the original conditioned stimulus is no longer associated with danger. Theoretically, estrogen treatment in a patient with panic disorder may enhance the deconditioning or extinction of panic reactions by facilitating the acquisition of alternative cognitive appraisals of anxiety or fear stimuli.

Progesterone

Progesterone administered alone has anxiolytic effects in several behavioral paradigms, including increased exploratory behavior in an elevated plus-maze and open field (Banerjee 1971; Mora et al. 1996) and reduced conditioned avoidance (Diaz-Veliz et al. 1994; Farr et al. 1995). Reductions in fear behaviors in response to progesterone have been attributed to potentiation of $GABA_A$ receptors, the same receptors activated by the benzodiazepines, but may also involve co-modulation with estrogen of other neurotransmitter and neuropeptide systems.

There has been little formal study of the effects of progesterone administration on anxiety disorders in humans. The animal and preclinical literature suggests that clinical trials of progesterone or anxiolytic progesterone metabolites or neurosteroids are warranted in patients with anxiety disorders. Although beneficial effects of progesterone on several premenstrual symptoms, including anxiety, were initially reported, these findings were not confirmed in controlled trials. On the contrary, after induction of a hypogonadal state via administration of a depot luteinizing hormone–releasing hormone agonist, progesterone administration was shown to exacerbate premenstrual syndrome symptoms in women with a history of premenstrual syndrome and to have no effect on mood in healthy women undergoing the same hormonal treatment regimen (Schmidt et al. 1998). Again, these data indicate that some women with psychiatric disorders are likely to have a differential sensitivity to gonadal steroids.

Androgens

As previously mentioned, the effects of androgenic steroids are often mediated by estrogen receptors after testosterone is converted by local aromatase enzymes. However, androgen receptors are present in the brain and have been shown to have behavioral effects. Naturalistic and controlled studies of testosterone administration in men indicate that aggressive and manic behavior occur only at supraphysiological dosages (600 mg testosterone per week) and that only some individuals are vulnerable to developing these effects (Pope and Katz, in press).

Although open studies have suggested that inhibition of androgen production via administration of cyproterone acetate or spironolactone and testolactone can ameliorate OCD symptoms (Casas et al. 1986; Leonard 1989), this effect does not seem to be mediated through androgen receptors, since treatment of OCD patients with flutamide, a specific androgen receptor antagonist, was not beneficial in another study (Altemus et al., in press). Apparently, relief of OCD symptoms during inhibition of androgen production is attributable to decreased stimulation of estrogen receptors rather than to a direct effect on androgen receptors. Worsening of OCD through estrogen receptor activation is consistent with reports of onset and worsening of OCD during pregnancy (Nezeroglu et al. 1992) and with the equal prevalence of the disorder in males and females (i.e., if androgen receptors were involved, one would expect the illness to be much more common in men than in women). Interestingly, high levels of the neuropeptides oxytocin and vasopressin have been linked to OCD (Altemus 1995; Leckman et al. 1994). Activity of both of these neuropeptides is profoundly stimulated by estrogen (DeVries et al. 1994; McCarthy 1995).

Estrus Cycle/Menstrual Cycle

Behavior changes noted across the estrus cycle reflect an interaction of estrogen and progesterone effects. In the estrus cycle of most species, estrogen rises first, then progesterone rises, initially potentiating but then, after 6–12 hours, antagonizing the effects of estrogen. In the 4- to 5-day rat estrus cycle, estrogen peaks in early proestrus, progesterone peaks in late proestrus, and both reach a nadir in metestrus.

Because many different hormones fluctuate with the estrus cycle, it is often difficult to gauge the influence of a particular gonadal steroid on a biological mechanism or behavior. However, it is also not adequate to examine the behavioral effects of estrogen and progesterone only in isolation. Estrogen upregulates progesterone receptors in many brain areas (Parsons et al. 1982). Because of this, many progesterone effects on behavior—for example, lordosis induction and reduced locomotion—can be seen only after estrogen priming (Rodier 1971).

In the rat, many behavioral effects of estrogen, including inhibition of avoidance behavior, have been shown to peak at 24–48 hours after exogenous estrogen dosing (Diaz-Veliz et al. 1989). This 48-hour lag before peak behavioral effect suggests that estrogen is working through genomic rather than nongenomic mechanisms. In the natural estrus cycle, however, the anxiolytic effects of estrogen are shorter in duration than those induced by exogenous estrogen dosing, presumably because of progesterone antagonism of estrogen effects. Consistent with this model, in most behavioral paradigms, measures of fear behavior are reduced in proestrus and estrus only, up to 24 hours after circulating estrogen rises, compared with metestrus and diestrus, when progesterone antagonism of estrogen effects has come into play. During proestrus and estrus, rats showed less defensive behavior after a shock probe was introduced into the cage (Fernandez-Guasti and Picazo 1990), increased activity in an open field (Anderson 1940; Burke and Broadhurst 1966; A. Gray and Levine 1964), slower acquisition of avoidance responses to footshock (Farr et al. 1995), and predominantly increased entrance into the open arms of the plus-maze (Bitran et al. 1991; Diaz-Veliz et al.

1997; Mora et al. 1996; Nomikos and Spiraki 1988). Also, in proestrus, female rats appear to be more sensitive to the anxiolytic effect of diazepam (Fernandez-Guasti and Picazo 1990), suggesting that similar changes in benzodiazepine sensitivity may occur across the menstrual cycle in humans.

Of note, female rats show a reduction in conditioned freezing, a measure of anxiety, only on the afternoon of proestrus, as compared with the morning of proestrus and estrus (Markus and Zecevic 1997), a finding that implicates elevated levels of circulating estrogen as a mechanism. The relatively rapid shift in this measure of fear, compared with the persistence of anxiolytic effects throughout proestrus and estrus in other animal models of anxiety, suggests that the mechanism by which estrogen influences this behavior is nongenomic.

Two studies have indicated that the anxiolytic effects of progesterone may be seen only in estrogen-primed rats. Acute injections of progesterone (5 hours before testing) in estrogen-primed rats (daily estrogen injections for 5 days) have been shown to increase punished responding (i.e., drinking from a bottle that delivers shock) in females (Rodriguez-Sierra 1984; Rodriguez-Sierra et al. 1986). This effect was not seen with either hormone administered individually.

In contrast to the 4- to 5-day estrus cycle in the rat, in humans the sequential rise in estrogen and progesterone occurs over a much longer period (4 weeks). Thus, unopposed behavioral effects of estrogen should be present up to and including the early luteal phase of the cycle, and progesterone antagonism of estrogen effects should occur in the midluteal phase, followed by a loss of estrogen and progesterone in the late luteal phase. Thus, if estrogen has anxiolytic effects in humans, as seen in rats, these effects should be evident in the follicular and early luteal phases of the cycle and should be lost in the latter half of the luteal phase. Indirect support for this model in humans comes from evidence that the mood-lifting effects of estrogen in postmenopausal women are often lost during periods of progesterone co-administration (Zweifel and O'Brien 1997) and that women with premenstrual dysphoric disorder commonly experience increased anxiety during the late luteal phase of the cycle (Rubinow and Roy-Byrne 1984).

Pregnancy

In addition to varying with the estrus cycle, gonadal hormones vary with other reproductive events as well. Pregnancy is characterized by steep rises in both estrogens and progestogens, whereas the postpartum period is characterized by a dramatic decrease in these steroids with the termination of gestation. There has been relatively little study in females of the behavioral and brain effects of androstenedione, dehydroepiandrosterone (DHEA), and other adrenal androgens, levels of which also increase markedly during pregnancy and during the luteal phase of the menstrual cycle.

One retrospective study and several case series have pointed toward a reduction in panic disorder symptoms during pregnancy in humans (Klein et al. 1995). In contrast, a number of case series and a retrospective study of OCD reported an increase in symptom severity during pregnancy (Altshuler et al. 1998; Nezeroglu et al. 1992). The differential course of these two disorders during pregnancy could be related to several factors. Increased cerebrospinal fluid (CSF) GABA levels have been described in sheep during pregnancy (Kendrick et al. 1988b), and high progesterone levels during pregnancy are likely to facilitate transmission at $GABA_A$ receptors. GABA agonists are very effective in treating panic but provide little relief of OCD symptoms. In addition, rising gonadal steroid levels during pregnancy may reduce serotonergic activity, an effect that may be more harmful in patients with OCD than in patients with panic disorder.

Pregnancy can also precipitate the development of anxiety through pregnancy-related alterations in immune function. Antithyroid antibodies are present in 10%–20% of women of childbearing age. Although these antibodies are usually nonpathological, studies have shown that titers become markedly elevated postpartum (Solomon et al. 1993) and that women with antithyroid antibodies are at greatly increased risk of autoimmune thyroiditis. Postpartum thyroiditis may cause an increase in thyroid hormone production during the first several months postpartum. This condition often evolves into hypothyroidism later in the first year postpartum (Solomon et al. 1993). Hyperthyroidism is well known to produce anxiety symptoms, and hypothyroidism can lead to depression.

Lactation

Lactation in all mammalian species is associated with a unique endocrine repertoire characterized by enhanced episodic secretion of oxytocin and prolactin and suppression of the HPA axis (McNeilly et al. 1994). In addition, a series of studies in lactating rats have demonstrated that lactation is accompanied by consistent reductions in the usual endocrine responses to stress. Findings in lactating rats include reductions in plasma adrenocorticotropin (Lightman 1992; Walker et al. 1992), corticosterone (Lightman 1992; Walker et al. 1992), catecholamine (Higuchi et al. 1989), and prolactin (Higuchi et al. 1989; Pohl et al. 1989) responses to physical stressors. Lactating rats also show significant decreases in several CNS responses to stress, including hippocampal immediate early gene induction (Abbud et al. 1992), hypothalamic CRH messenger RNA (mRNA) production (Lightman and Young 1989), and expression of fear behaviors (Fleming and Luebke 1981; Hansen and Ferreira 1986).

In healthy humans, lactation also suppresses hormonal response to exercise stress (Altemus et al. 1995) and autonomic nervous system response to distressed infant cries (Weisenfeld et al. 1985). In women with panic disorder, lactation seems to have a protective effect, with panic symptoms recurring after weaning. A retrospective study of a large group of mothers with panic disorder showed a dramatic reduction of panic attack frequency, but not of agoraphobia, during pregnancy and lactation (Klein et al. 1995).

The exact physiological mechanisms mediating the reduction in stress response in lactating women and animals remain to be clarified. Increased levels of GABA have been reported in the CSF of lactating rats (Qureshi et al. 1987). Studies in sheep and rats show that oxytocin, a neuropeptide with anxiolytic properties (McCarthy and Altemus 1997), is released during lactation into the CSF and into several brain areas (Kendrick et al. 1986, 1988a; Neumann and Landgraf 1989). One study that examined intrathecal oxytocin administration in humans with back pain found an analgesic effect (Yang 1994). Production of neuropeptide Y, another neuropeptide with anxiolytic properties, is also greatly enhanced during lactation (M. S. Smith 1993).

Lactation-induced suppression of fear behaviors, the HPA axis, and autonomic arousal may have several adaptive functions for both the mother and her infant. First, conservation of energy needed for synthesis of milk would be promoted both by reduced tonic sympathetic outflow and by inhibition of HPA axis activation and the associated catabolic effects of glucocorticoid secretion. Second, inhibition of CRH and catecholamine release could minimize psychological arousal or anxiety associated with the demands of infant care, thereby potentially facilitating maternal behaviors. Third, reduced psychological reactivity during lactation could attenuate the reductions in milk release known to occur with stress (Newton and Newton 1948). Although prolactin has also been shown to blunt hormonal responses to stress in animals (Endroczi and Nyakas 1972; Schlein et al. 1974), the nonreproductive behavioral effects of prolactin have received little attention.

Sex Differences in Animal Anxiety Models

Although women are clearly more prone than are men to developing panic disorder, PTSD, and phobias, studies of sex differences in fear behaviors have produced mixed results that seem to vary among different strains of rats. In two studies (Maren et al. 1994; Markus and Zecevic 1997), female rats have been shown to exhibit reduced fear behavior in a contextual fear–conditioning task but not a cued fear–conditioning task. In another conditioned avoidance paradigm, male rats again demonstrated stronger conditioned avoidance of a footshock than did females (Farr et al. 1995). In addition, in the learned helplessness model, male rats exhibited impaired avoidance conditioning after exposure to inescapable shock, but this effect of inescapable shock was much less evident in females (Heinsbroek et al. 1991).

Generally increased activity levels in females compared with males, and sex differences in a variety of other behavioral parameters, including information processing, pain sensitivity, and appetite, complicate interpretation of sex differences in animal models of anxiety. In addition, findings of sex differences may be the result of more consistent state-dependent learning in males (Markus and Zecevic 1997). That is, female rats may be less likely to recall a fear association if it is learned while the rat is in one hormonal state but reexposure occurs during a different hormonal state. Findings in earlier studies that female rats had impaired learned avoidance behavior may have been the result of training and testing females in different parts of their estrus cycles.

Sexually Dimorphic Impact of Stress on Behavior and Neural Structure

Although sex differences in HPA axis responsivity have been well described, sex differences in extrahypothalamic and behavioral responses to stress have only recently come to light. Perhaps most surprising, there are sex differences in the impact of stress on performance of a number of learned behaviors, including classical conditioning, operant conditioning, and conditioned fear behaviors. In male rats, stress is well known to facilitate classical conditioning of behaviors such as eye blinking when an air puff to the eye is paired with a tone signal. In female rats, however, stress impairs acquisition of eye-blink conditioning. This sex difference appears to be estrogen dependent, since impairment of conditioning in females could be abolished by ovariectomy or treatment with an estrogen receptor antagonist and restored in ovariectomized rats by estrogen treatment (Wood and Shors 1998). In male but not female rats, exposure to inescapable shock reduced subsequent movement into the open arm of an elevated plus-maze and shuttlebox-escape performance (Kirk and Blampied 1985; Steenbergen et al. 1990). Female rats likewise showed a smaller magnitude of behavior changes after exposure to a restraint stress, but also exhibited a failure of behavioral adaptation to repeated restraint stress, indicating that their behavioral reactivity to stress was more persistent than that of males (Kennet et al. 1986).

Another striking finding is that the acute effects of stress on neural structure are also sexually dimorphic. Although exposure to chronic stress over 21 days produced atrophy of apical dendrites of CA3 hippocampal pyramidal neurons in male rats, this effect was not seen in females (Galea et al. 1997). In a related study, repeated swim stress over 30 days decreased CA3 and CA4 pyramidal cell numbers in gonadectomized male rats but not in female rats (Mizoguchi et al. 1992). Similar results were found in a study of chronic stress in male and female vervet monkeys (Uno et al. 1989). The reduced amount of hippocampal atrophy found in females is particularly surprising in light of the prolonged corticosterone responsivity noted in females compared with males in multiple acute and chronic stress studies (Galea et al. 1997) and in view of evidence that corticosterone mediates CA3 dendritic atrophy (Jacobson and Sapolsky 1991; Mafarinos and McEwen 1995). These findings raise the possibility that women may be relatively protected from the hippocampal atrophy associated with elevated cortisol levels in humans with Cushing's syndrome (Starkman et al. 1992) and depression (Sheline et al. 1996), as well as the hippocampal atrophy associated with increased glucocorticoid receptor sensitivity in PTSD (Bremner et al. 1995; Yehuda et al. 1995).

There is also evidence of sex differences in developmental responses to prenatal stress. Prenatal stress results in exaggerated stress responses across several dimensions in adulthood, including increased emotional reactivity, increased anxiety-associated behaviors, and reduced numbers of hippocampal glucocorticoid receptors. Compared with prenatally stressed males, as adults, prenatally stressed females have increased HPA axis responsivity and greater reductions in glucocorticoid receptor binding in the amygdala and septum (McCormick et al. 1995). This suggests that prenatal stress has a more profound effect in females than in males on later HPA axis regulation. Similarly, perinatal manipulation of gonadal steroid hormones has been found to permanently alter several components of brain stress response systems, including glucocorticoid receptor binding, hypothalamic CRH and vasopressin gene expression, and HPA axis responsivity to estradiol (Patchev et al. 1995). Unfortunately, fear-associated behaviors were not examined in these studies of sex differences in the sequelae of prenatal and perinatal stress.

Effects of Gonadal Steroids on Selected Anxiety-Related Neurochemical Systems

The biological mechanisms underlying these divergent responses to stress in males and females are unclear. Studies to date indicate that sexual differentiation during development contributes to these sex differences in stress responsivity, and that acute effects of gonadal steroid hormones on multiple neurotransmitter systems also appear to play an important role.

Glucocorticoids

One mechanism underlying sex differences in stress responsivity is interactions between gonadal steroids and glucocorticoid hormones and receptors. Evidence indicates that estrogen and progesterone may antagonize the actions of stress by antagonizing glucocorticoid activity. A gonadal steroid antagonism of glucocorticoid activity could be extremely important, given that exogenous glucocorticoids and stress-induced release of glucocorticoids have been shown to play a critical role in generating the behavioral and biological pathophysiology of anxiety. Glucocorticoids potentiate anxiety in animal models (Corodimas et al. 1994; Roozendaal and McGaugh 1996) and are associated with memory impairment in animals and humans (Starkman et al. 1992). Glucocorticoids also have been shown to decrease serotonergic receptor expression in the hippocampus (Lopez et al. 1998) and to increase activity of CRH in the amygdala and bed nucleus of the stria terminalis (Makino et al. 1994; Watts and Sanchez-Watts 1995), two other systems that have been closely linked to fear behaviors and physiological responses to stress. Interference with glucocorticoid activity may occur through antagonism or downregulation of glucocorticoid receptors (Burgess and Handa 1992) or through interference with the nuclear function of ligand-bound glucocorticoid receptors (Uht et al. 1997). Progesterone can act as a glucocorticoid antagonist and, like estrogen, may potentially counteract the effects of stress-induced release of glucocorticoids (Keller-Wood et al. 1988; Svec et al.

1980). Androgens also appear to inhibit some effects of gluco-corticoids through competition for receptor binding (Mayer and Rosen 1975) and through interactions of the activated hormone-bound receptors prior to binding to transcription sites (Chen et al. 1997).

Serotonin

Gonadal steroids also are likely to modulate anxiety through effects on serotonergic systems. (Effects of estrogen on seroto-nergic transmission are reviewed in Chapter 5 of this volume.) Overall, the literature suggests that estrogen enhances the effi-ciency of serotonergic neurotransmission. No consistent effects of progesterone administration on serotonin function have been identified. However, limited evidence suggests that like estro-gen, progesterone may upregulate $5\text{-}HT_2$ receptors (Biegon et al. 1983) and increase serotonin synthesis (Pecins-Thompson et al. 1996). There also is evidence that testosterone's effects on seroto-nergic activity are opposite to those of estrogen and progester-one. Reductions in androgenic steroids have been associated with enhancement of brain serotonergic activity (Bonson et al. 1994; Fischette et al. 1984; Matsuda et al. 1991). In addition, ad-ministration of testosterone has been associated with reductions in brain serotonergic activity (Martinez-Conde et al. 1985; Mendelson and McEwen 1990). Of note, the two illnesses shown to have a specific response to serotonergic antidepressants, pre-menstrual syndrome (Eriksson et al. 1995) and OCD (Greist et al. 1995), appear to be particularly sensitive to changes in gonadal steroids.

Glutamate

Another factor that may contribute to sex differences in the stress response is reproductive hormone–related changes in glutama-tergic activity. Glutamate is the primary excitatory transmitter in the brain. Activation of the glutamatergic system triggers anxiety, long-term potentiation (an electrophysiological animal model of learning), and seizures. Estrogen activation of both the NMDA and the non-NMDA types of glutamate receptors (Gazzaley et al. 1996; S. S. Smith 1989; Weiland 1992a; Wong and Moss 1992) is likely to contribute to estrogen- and proestrus-associated reductions in the seizure threshold (Buterbaugh and Hudson 1991; Terasawa and Timiras 1967; Teyler et al. 1980) and to increases in long-term potentiation during proestrus and estrogen treatment (Warren et al. 1995; Wong and Moss 1992). These changes in seizure threshold and long-term potentiation are consistent with observations of increases in synaptic density and in the number of dendritic spines in the CA1 nucleus of the hippocampus during estrogen treatment and during proestrus (Woolley and McEwen 1992). NMDA receptor activation is known to underlie estrogen-induced increases in synaptic density in the CA3 region of the hippocampus (Woolley and McEwen 1994). These effects of estrogen on glutamatergic transmission appear to involve genomic as well as nongenomic mechanisms.

However, estrogen potentiation of glutamatergic receptors does not at first seem consistent with estrogen-associated reductions in anxiety, given that glutamate agonists promote a variety of fear behaviors. Interestingly, although estrogen treatment reduces the seizure threshold in the hippocampus and the medial amygdala, it raises the seizure threshold in the lateral nucleus of the amygdala (Terasawa and Timiras 1967), which, unlike the medial amygdala, plays an important role in generation of conditioned and unconditioned fear behaviors (LeDoux 1996). These discordant effects suggest a mechanism whereby estrogen may enhance memory but also decrease anxiety. Another mechanism contributing to this inverse relationship between the hippocampus and the lateral amygdala in seizure threshold versus fear behavior may be tonic inhibition of amygdala activity by the hippocampus (J. A. Gray 1982). Rats with bilateral hippocampal lesions demonstrate several fear-associated behaviors, including enhanced acquisition of conditioned avoidance (Pitman 1982; Port et al. 1991) and delayed extinction of conditioned responses (Devenport 1978; Schmaltz and Isaacson 1967).

Gamma-Aminobutyric Acid

The amino acid GABA, synthesized from glutamate, is the dominant inhibitory neurotransmitter in the brain. The $GABA_A$ subtype of GABA receptor is widely distributed in the CNS, primarily postsynaptically, and inhibits neuronal firing by opening a Cl^- channel. The $GABA_A$ receptor, the benzodiazepine binding site, and the Cl^- ionophore are part of a single large macromolecular complex. A number of progesterone metabolites or neurosteroids potentiate GABA activity by binding to the $GABA_A$ receptor.

Estrogen also has multiple effects on GABA systems, consistent with its production of anxiolytic effects. Estrogen has been shown to increase GABA receptor binding in the hippocampus (Schumacher et al. 1989). Finally, production of mRNA for glutamic acid decarboxylase, the rate-limiting enzyme for GABA synthesis, is enhanced in the hippocampus (Weiland 1992b) and the midbrain (McCarthy et al. 1995b) during estrogen treatment. Progesterone administered alone had no effect on GABA receptor binding (Schumacher et al. 1989) but, when co-administered with estrogen, reversed the estrogen-induced increase in hippocampal glutamic acid decarboxylase mRNA (Weiland 1992b).

The observation that activity in an open field in response to diazepam is enhanced in estrogen-treated rats (McCarthy et al. 1995a) is consistent with these neurobiological studies and suggests that estrogen may increase sensitivity to benzodiazepine treatment in humans.

Conclusion

The bulk of evidence from animal studies suggests that, at least in females, reproductive hormones limit expression of behavioral stress and fear responses. This modulation of anxiety by reproductive hormones may actually represent a high-order, integrative aspect of reproductive physiology. Although the brain systems critical to reproductive behaviors are to a large degree distinct from those implicated in the generation of anxiety and fear, limitation of anxiety may be a necessary condition for performance of sexual and social behaviors. Reduced anxiety during proestrus or during the midcycle phase in humans may increase exposure to possible mates by decreasing fear of novel or otherwise threatening environments and social contacts (Carter and Altemus 1997; McCarthy et al. 1996). In addition, reduced anxiety during lactation should facilitate milk release and maternal care in general.

These animal data parallel emerging clinical observations of anxiolytic and antidepressant effects of estrogen and progesterone. On the other hand, clinical data also suggest that some reproductive hormones, particularly estrogen and androgens, may potentiate psychiatric symptoms in some individuals. Because the gonadal steroids have so many effects on multiple brain systems, effects of these hormones are likely to vary among individuals on the basis of underlying differences in target neurochemical systems. For example, women with low serotonin levels or low serotonergic neurotransmission may experience increases rather than decreases in anxiety and irritability during the premenstrual phase of the cycle, as progesterone antagonizes a proserotonergic effect of estrogen and then estrogen levels also drop. Future studies with inbred rat strains may identify strains with similar, paradoxical behavioral responses to estrogen and progesterone.

The fact that women experience much greater and repetitive fluctuations in reproductive hormones over the life span may enhance the potential for dysregulation of a wide variety of brain neurochemical systems, likely contributing to the enhanced vulnerability to depression and anxiety disorders in women. Dysregulation of glucocorticoid, serotonergic, and glutamatergic systems may be particularly important in potentiating the development of these disorders. New data indicate that there are multiple levels of interaction among glucocorticoid hormones released in response to stress and the gonadal steroids.

Future work with animal behavioral models and continued examination of the effects of reproductive hormones on brain structure and function should further enhance our understanding of the pathophysiology of anxiety disorders in both men and women and lead to new treatment approaches.

References

Abbud R, Lee WS, Hoffman GE, et al: Lactation inhibits hippocampal and cortical activation of c-*fos* expression by NMDA but not kainate receptor agonists. Mol Cell Neurosci 3:244–250, 1992

Albeck D, McKittrick CR, Blanchard DC, et al: Chronic social stress alters levels of corticotropin-releasing factor and arginine vasopressin mRNA in rat brain. J Neurosci 17:4895–4903, 1997

Altemus M: Neuroendocrinology of obsessive-compulsive disorder. Advances in Biological Psychiatry 1:215–233, 1995

Altemus M, Pigott T, Kalogeras KT, et al: Abnormalities in the regulation of vasopressin and corticotropin releasing factor secretion in obsessive-compulsive disorder. Arch Gen Psychiatry 49:9–20, 1992

Altemus M, Deuster P, Galliven E, et al: Suppression of hypothalamic-pituitary-adrenal axis responses to stress in lactating women. J Clin Endocrinol Metab 80:2954–2959, 1995

Altemus M, Conrad CD, Dolan S, et al: Estrogen reduces fear conditioning: differential effects on context vs. tone conditioning (abstract). Biol Psychiatry 43:14S, 1998

Altemus M, Greenberg BD, Keuler D, et al: Open trial of flutamide for treatment of obsessive-compulsive disorder. J Clin Psychiatry (in press)

Altshuler LL, Hendrick V, Cohen LS: Course of mood and anxiety disorders during pregnancy and the postpartum period. J Clin Psychiatry 59 (suppl 12):29–33, 1998

Anderson EE: The sex hormones and emotional behavior, I: the effect of sexual receptivity upon timidity in the female rat. J Genet Psychol 56:149–158, 1940

Auricchio F: Phosphorylation of steroid receptors. Journal of Steroid Biochemistry 32:613–622, 1989

Banerjee U: Influence of pseudopregnancy and sex hormones on conditioned behavior in rats. Neuroendocrinology 7:278–290, 1971

Biegon A, Reches A, Snyder L, et al: Serotonergic and noradrenergic receptors in the rat brain: modulation by chronic exposure to ovarian hormones. Life Sci 32:2015–2021, 1983

Bitran D, Hilvers RJ, Kellogg CK: Ovarian endocrine status modulates the anxiolytic potency of diazepam and the efficacy of gamma-aminobutyric acid–benzodiazepine receptor-mediated chloride ion transport. Behav Neurosci 105:652–662, 1991

Bonson KR, Johnson RG, Fiorella D, et al: Serotonergic control of androgen-induced dominance. Pharmacol Biochem Behav 49:313–322, 1994

Brady L, Whitfield HJ, Fox RJ, et al: Long-term antidepressant administration alters corticotropin releasing hormone, tyrosine hydroxylase and mineralocorticoid receptor gene expression in rat brain: therapeutic implications. J Clin Invest 87:831–837, 1991

Breier A, Davis O, Buchanan R, et al: Effects of alprazolam on pituitary-adrenal and catecholaminergic responses to metabolic stress in humans. Biol Psychiatry 15:880–890, 1992

Bremner JD, Randall P, Scott TM, et al: MRI-based measurement of hippocampal volume in patients with combat-related posttraumatic stress disorder. Am J Psychiatry 152:973–981, 1995

Bremner JD, Licinio J, Darnell A, et al: Elevated CSF corticotropin-releasing factor concentrations in post-traumatic stress disorder. Am J Psychiatry 154:624–629, 1997

Burgess LH, Handa RJ: Chronic estrogen-induced alterations in adrenocorticotropin and corticosterone secretion, and glucocorticoid receptor-mediated functions in female rats. Endocrinology 131:1261–1269, 1992

Burke AW, Broadhurst PL: Behavioral correlates of the oestrous cycle in the rat. Nature 209:223–224, 1966

Buterbaugh GG, Hudson GM: Estradiol replacement to female rats facilitates dorsal hippocampal but not ventral hippocampal kindled seizure acquisition. Exp Neurol 111:55–64, 1991

Carter CS, Altemus M: Integrative function of lactational hormones in social behavior and stress management. Ann N Y Acad Sci 807:164–174, 1997

Casas M, Alvarez E, Duro P, et al: Antiandrogenic treatment of obsessive-compulsive neurosis. Acta Psychiatr Scand 73:221–222, 1986

Charney D, Woods S, Goodman W, et al: Neurobiological mechanisms of panic anxiety: biochemical and behavioral correlates of yohimbine-induced panic attacks. Am J Psychiatry 144:1030–1036, 1987

Chen Sy, Wang J, Yu Gq, et al: Androgen and glucocorticoid receptor heterodimer formation: a possible mechanism for mutual inhibition of transcriptional activity. J Biol Chem 272:14087–14092, 1997

Chrousos GP, Gold PW: The concepts of stress and stress system disorders: overview of physical and behavioral homeostasis. JAMA 267:1244–1252, 1992

Coplan JD, Andrews MW, Rosenblum LA, et al: Persistent elevations of cerebrospinal fluid concentrations of corticotropin-releasing factor in adult nonhuman primates exposed to early life stressors: implications for the pathophysiology of mood and anxiety disorders. Proc Natl Acad Sci U S A 93:1619–1623, 1996

Corodimas KP, LeDoux JE, Gold PW, et al: Corticosterone potentiation of learned fear. Ann N Y Acad Sci 746:392–393, 1994

Devenport LD: Schedule-induced polydipsia in rats: adrenocortical and hippocampal modulation. Journal of Comparative and Physiological Psychology 92:651–660, 1978

DeVries GJ, Wang Z, Bullock NA: Sex differences in the effects of testosterone and its metabolites on vasopressin messenger RNA levels in the bed nucleus of the stria terminalis of rats. J Neurosci 14:1789–1794, 1994

Diaz-Veliz G, Soto V, Dussaubat N, et al: Influence of the estrous cycle, ovariectomy and estradiol replacement upon the acquisition of conditioned avoidance responses in rats. Physiol Behav 46:397–401, 1989

Diaz-Veliz G, Urresta F, Dussaubat N, et al: Effects of estradiol replacement in ovariectomized rats on conditioned avoidance responses and other behaviors. Physiol Behav 50:61–65, 1991

Diaz-Veliz G, Urresta F, Dussaubat N, et al: Progesterone effects on the acquisition of conditioned avoidance responses and other motoric behaviors in intact and ovariectomized rats. Psychoneuroendocrinology 19:387–394, 1994

Diaz-Veliz G, Alarcon T, Espinoza C, et al: Ketanserin and anxiety level: influence of gender, estrus cycle, ovariectomy and ovarian hormones in female rats. Pharmacol Biochem Behav 58:637–642, 1997

Ditkoff EC, Crary WG, Cristo M, et al: Estrogen improves psychological function in asymptomatic postmenopausal women. Obstet Gynecol 78:991–995, 1991

Dohanich GP, Fader AJ, Javorsky DJ: Estrogen and estrogen–progesterone treatments counteract the effect of scopolamine on reinforced T-maze alternation in female rats. Behav Neurosci 108:988–992, 1994

Drugan RC, Maier SF, Skolnick P, et al: An anxiogenic benzodiazepine receptor ligand induced learned helplessness. Eur J Pharmacol 113:453–457, 1985

elMansari M, Bouchard C, Blier P: Alteration of serotonin release in the guinea pig orbitofrontal cortex by selective serotonin reuptake inhibitors: relevance to treatment of obsessive-compulsive disorder. Neuropsychopharmacology 13:117–127, 1995

Endroczi E, Nyakas CS: Pituitary adrenal function during lactation and after LTH (prolactin) administration in the rat. Acta Physiologica Academiae Scientiarum Hungaricae 41:49–54, 1972

Eriksson E, Hedberg MA, Andersch B, et al: The serotonin reuptake inhibitor paroxetine is superior to the noradrenaline reuptake inhibitor maprotiline in the treatment of premenstrual syndrome. Neuropsychopharmacology 12:167–176, 1995

Farr SA, Flood JF, Scherrer JF, et al: Effect of ovarian steroids on foot-shock avoidance learning and retention in female mice. Physiol Behav 58:715–723, 1995

Fernandez-Guasti A, Picazo O: The actions of diazepam and seroto-nergic anxiolytics vary according to the gender and the estrous cycle phase. Pharmacol Biochem Behav 37:77–81, 1990

Fischette CT, Biegon A, McEwen BS: Sex steroid modulation of the se-rotonin behavioral syndrome. Life Sci 35:1197–1206, 1984

Fleming AS, Luebke C: Timidity prevents the virgin female rat from be-ing a good mother: emotionality differences between nulliparous and parturient females. Physiol Behav 27:863–868, 1981

Galea LM, McEwen BS, Tanapat P, et al: Sex differences in dendritic at-rophy of CA3 pyramidal neurons in response to chronic restraint stress. Neuroscience 81:689–697, 1997

Gazzaley AH, Weiland NG, McEwen BS, et al: Differential regulation of NMDAR1 mRNA and protein by estradiol in the rat hippocam-pus. J Neurosci 16:6830–6838, 1996

Gold PW, Goodwin FK, Chrousos GP: Clinical and biochemical mani-festations of depression: relation to the neurobiology of stress. N Engl J Med 319:413–420, 1988

Gray A, Levine S: Effect of induced oestrus on emotional behaviour in selected strains of rats. Nature 201:1198–1200, 1964

Gray JA: The Neuropsychology of Anxiety: An Enquiry into the Func-tioning of the Septohippocampal System. New York, Oxford Uni-versity Press, 1982

Greist JH, Jefferson JW, Kobak KA, et al: Efficacy and tolerability of se-rotonin transport inhibitors in obsessive-compulsive disorder. Arch Gen Psychiatry 52:53–60, 1995

Hansen S, Ferreira A: Food intake, aggression and fear behavior in the mother rat: control by neural systems concerned with milk ejection and maternal behavior. Behav Neurosci 100:410–415, 1986

Heim C, Owens MJ, Plotsky PM, et al: Persistent changes in cortico-tropin-releasing factor systems due to early life stress: relationship to the pathophysiology of major depression and post-traumatic stress disorder. Psychopharmacol Bull 33:185–192, 1997

Heinsbroek R, Haaren FV, Van der Poll N, et al: Sex differences in the behavioral consequences of inescapable footshocks depend on time since shock. Physiol Behav 49:1257–1263, 1991

Heninger GR, Charney DS: Mechanism of action of antidepressant treatment: implications for the etiology and treatment of depressive disorders, in Psychopharmacology: The Third Generation of Prog-ress. Edited by Meltzer HY. New York, Raven, 1987, pp 535–544

Henn FA, McKinney WT: Animal models in psychiatry, in Psychopharmacology: The Third Generation of Progress. Edited by Meltzer HY. New York, Raven, 1987, pp 687–696

Higuchi T, Negoro H, Arita J: Reduced responses of prolactin and catecholamine to stress in the lactating rat. J Endocrinol 122:495–498, 1989

Jacobson L, Sapolsky R: The role of the hippocampus in feedback regulation of the hypothalamic-pituitary-adrenocortical axis. Endocr Rev 12:118–134, 1991

Kampen DL, Sherwin BB: Estrogen use and verbal memory in healthy postmenopausal women. Obstet Gynecol 83:979–983, 1994

Katzenellenbogen JA, O'Malley BW, Katzenellenbogen BS: Tripartite steroid hormone receptor pharmacology: interaction with multiple effector sites as a basis for the cell- and promoter-specific action of these hormones. Mol Endocrinol 10:119–131, 1996

Keller-Wood M, Silbiger J, Wood CE: Progesterone attenuates the inhibition of adrenocorticotropin responses by cortisol in nonpregnant ewes. Endocrinology 123:647–651, 1988

Kendler KS: Major depression and generalised anxiety disorder: same genes, (partly) different environments—revisited. Br J Psychiatry Suppl 30:68–75, 1996

Kendrick KM, Keverne EB, Baldwin BA, et al: Cerebrospinal fluid levels of acetylcholinesterase, monoamines and oxytocin during labour, parturition, vaginocervical stimulation, lamb separation and suckling in sheep. Neuroendocrinology 44:149–156, 1986

Kendrick KM, Keverne EB, Chapman C, et al: Intracranial dialysis measurement of oxytocin, monoamine and uric acid release from the olfactory bulb and substantia nigra of sheep during parturition, suckling, separation from lambs and eating. Brain Res 439:1–10, 1988a

Kendrick KM, Keverne EB, Chapman C, et al: Microdialysis measurement of oxytocin, aspartate, gamma-aminobutyric acid and glutamate release from the olfactory bulb of the sheep during vaginocervical stimulation. Brain Res 442:171–174, 1988b

Kennet G, Chaouloff F, Marcou M, et al: Female rats are more vulnerable than males in an animal model of depression: the possible role of serotonin. Brain Res 382:416–421, 1986

Kirk RC, Blampied NM: Activity during inescapable shock and subsequent escape avoidance learning: females and males compared. New Zealand Journal of Psychology 14:9–14, 1985

Klein DF, Skrobala AM, Garfinkel RS: Preliminary look at the effects of pregnancy on the course of panic disorder. Anxiety 1:227–232, 1995

Kuiper GG, Carlsson B, Grandien K, et al: Comparison of the ligand binding specificity and transcript tissue distribution of estrogen receptors α and β. Endocrinology 138:863–870, 1997

Leckman JF, Goodman WK, North WG, et al: The role of central oxytocin in obsessive-compulsive disorder and related normal behavior. Psychoneuroendocrinology 19:723–749, 1994

LeDoux J: The Emotional Brain. New York, Simon & Schuster, 1996

Leonard HL: Drug treatment of obsessive-compulsive disorder, in Obsessive-Compulsive Disorder in Children and Adolescents. Edited by Rapoport JL. Washington, DC, American Psychiatric Press, 1989, pp 217–236

Lightman SL: Alterations in hypothalamic-pituitary responsiveness during lactation. Ann N Y Acad Sci 652:340–346, 1992

Lightman SL, Young WS: Lactation inhibits stress-mediated secretion of corticosterone and oxytocin and hypothalamic accumulation of corticotropin-releasing factor and enkephalin messenger ribonucleic acids. Endocrinology 124:2358–2364, 1989

Lindheim SR, Legro RS, Bernstein L, et al: Behavioral stress responses in premenopausal and postmenopausal women and the effects of estrogen. Am J Obstet Gynecol 167:1831–1836, 1992

Liu D, Diorio J, Tannenbaum B, et al: Maternal care, hippocampal glucocorticoid receptors, and hypothalamic-pituitary-adrenal responses to stress. Science 277:1659–1662, 1997

Lopez JF, Chalmers DT, Little KY, et al: Regulation of serotonin 1A, glucocorticoid, and mineralocorticoid receptor in rat and human hippocampus: implications for the neurobiology of depression. Biol Psychiatry 43:547–573, 1998

Luine VN: Steroid hormone influences on spatial memory. Ann N Y Acad Sci 743:201–211, 1994

Mafarinos AM, McEwen BS: Stress-induced atrophy of apical dendrites of hippocampal CA3c neurons: involvement of glucocorticosteroid secretion and excitatory amino acid receptors. Neuroscience 69:89–98, 1995

Maier SF, Seligman MEP: Learned helplessness: theory and evidence. Journal of Experimental Psychology 105:3–46, 1976

Makino S, Gold PW, Schulkin J: Effects of corticosterone on CRH mRNA and content in the bed nucleus of the stria terminalis: comparison with the effects in the central nucleus of the amygdala and the paraventricular nucleus of the hypothalamus. Brain Res 657: 141–149, 1994

Maren S, DeOc B, Fanselow MS: Sex differences in hippocampal long-term potentiation (LTP) and Pavlovian fear conditioning in rats: positive correlation between LTP and contextual learning. Brain Res 661:25–34, 1994

Markus EJ, Zecevic M: Sex differences and estrous cycle changes in hippocampus-dependent fear conditioning. Psychobiology 25:246–252, 1997

Martinez-Conde E, Leret ML, Diaz S: The influence of testosterone in the brain of the male rat on levels of serotonin (5-HT) and 5-hydroxyindoleacetic acid (5-HIAA). Comp Biochem Physiol C Pharmacol Toxicol Endocrinol 80:411–414, 1985

Matsuda T, Nakano Y, Kanda T, et al: Gonadal hormones affect the hypothermia induced by serotonin$_{1A}$ (5-HT$_{1A}$) receptor activation. Life Sci 48:1627–1632, 1991

Mayer M, Rosen F: Interaction of anabolic steroids with glucocorticoid receptor sites in rat muscle cytosol. Am J Physiol 229:1381–1386, 1975

McCarthy MM: Estrogen modulation of oxytocin and its relation to behavior, in Oxytocin. Edited by Ivell R, Russell J. New York, Plenum, 1995, pp 235–245

McCarthy MM, Altemus M: Central nervous system actions of oxytocin and modulation of behavior in humans. Mol Med Today (June):269–275, 1997

McCarthy MM, Felzenberg E, Robbins A, et al: Infusions of diazepam and allopregnenolone into the midbrain central gray facilitate open-field and reproductive behavior in female rats. Horm Behav 29:279–295, 1995a

McCarthy MM, Kaufman LC, Brooks PJ, et al: Estrogen modulation of mRNA levels for the two forms of glutamic acid decarboxylase (GAD) in female rat brain. J Comp Neurol 360:685–697, 1995b

McCarthy MM, Schwartz-Giblin S, Wang S: Does estrogen facilitate social behavior by reducing anxiety? Ann N Y Acad Sci 807:541–542, 1996

McCormick C, Smythe J, Sharma S, et al: Sex-specific effects of prenatal stress on hypothalamic-pituitary-adrenal responses to stress and brain glucocorticoid receptor density in adult rats. Brain Res Dev Brain Res 84:55–61, 1995

McEwen BS, Alves SE, Bulloch K, et al: Ovarian steroids and the brain: implications for cognition and aging. Neurology 48 (suppl 7):S8–S15, 1997

McNeilly AS, Tay CCK, Glasier A: Physiological mechanisms underlying lactational amenorrhea. Ann N Y Acad Sci 709:145–155, 1994

Mendelson SD, McEwen BA: Testosterone increases the concentration of (^{3}H)8-hydroxy-2-(di-n-propylamino)tetralin binding at 5-HT$_{1A}$ receptors in the medial preoptic nucleus of the castrated male rat. Eur J Pharmacol 181:329–331, 1990

Merikangas KR, Weissman MM, Pauls DL: Genetic factors in the sex ratio of major depression. Psychol Med 15:63–69, 1985

Meyer ME, Gronemeyer H, Turcotte B, et al: Steroid hormone receptors compete for factors that mediate their enhancer function. Cell 57:433–442, 1989

Mizoguchi K, Kunishita T, Chui DH, et al: Stress induces neuronal death in the hippocampus of castrated rats. Neurosci Lett 138:157–160, 1992

Mora S, Dussaubat N, Diaz-Veliz G: Effects of the estrous cycle and ovarian hormones on behavioral indices of anxiety in female rats. Psychoneuroendocrinology 21:609–620, 1996

Murua VS, Molina VA: Effects of chronic variable stress and antidepressant drugs on behavioral inactivity during an uncontrollable stress: interaction between both treatments. Behavioral and Neural Biology 57:87–89, 1992

Neumann I, Landgraf R: Septal and hippocampal release of oxytocin, but not vasopressin, in the conscious lactating rat during suckling. J Neuroendocrinol 1:305–308, 1989

Neumann ID, Johnstone HA, Hatzinger M, et al: Attenuated neuroendocrine responses to emotional and physical stressors in pregnant rats involve adenohypophysial changes. J Physiol (Lond) 508:289–300, 1998

Newton M, Newton NR: The let-down reflex in human lactation. J Pediatr 33:698–704, 1948

Nezeroglu F, Anemone R, Yaryura-Tobia J: Onset of obsessive-compulsive disorder in pregnancy. Am J Psychiatry 149:947–950, 1992

Nomikos GG, Spiraki C: Influence of oestrogen in spontaneous and diazepam-induced exploration of rats in an elevated plus-maze. Neuropharmacology 27:691–696, 1988

Ohkura T, Isse K, Akazewa K, et al: Long-term estrogen replacement therapy in female patients with dementia of the Alzheimer type: 7 case reports. Dementia 6:99–107, 1995

Packard MG, Teather LA: Posttraining estradiol injections enhance memory in ovariectomized rats: cholinergic blockade and synergism. Neurobiol Learn Mem 68:172–188, 1997

Paganini-Hill A, Henderson VW: Estrogen deficiency and risk of Alzheimer's disease in women. Am J Epidemiol 140:256–261, 1994

Parsons B, Rainbow TC, MacLusky NJ, et al: Progesterone receptor levels in rat hypothalamic and limbic nuclei. J Neurosci 2:1446–1452, 1982

Patchev V, Hayashi S, Orikasa C, et al: Implications of estrogen-dependent brain organization for gender difference in hypothalamic-pituitary-adrenal regulation. FASEB J 9:419–423, 1995

Pecins-Thompson M, Brown NA, Kohama SG, et al: Ovarian steroid regulation of tryptophan hydroxylase mRNA expression in rhesus macaques. J Neurosci 16:7021–7029, 1996

Pitman RK: Neurological etiology of obsessive-compulsive disorders? Am J Psychiatry 139:139–140, 1982

Pohl CR, Lee LR, Smith MS: Qualitative changes in luteinizing hormone and prolactin responses to N-methyl-D-aspartic acid during lactation in the rat. Endocrinology 124:1905–1911, 1989

Pope HG, Katz DL: Psychiatric effects of exogenous anabolic-androgenic steroids, in Psychoneuroendocrinology for the Clinician. Edited by Wolkowitz OM, Rothschild AJ. Washington, DC, American Psychiatric Press, in press

Port RL, Sample JA, Seybold KS: Partial hippocampal pyramidal cell loss alters behavior in rats: implications for an animal model of schizophrenia. Brain Res Bull 26:993–996, 1991

Prasad A, Imamura M, Prasad C: Dehydroepiandrosterone decreases behavioral despair in high- but not low-anxiety rats. Physiol Behav 62:1053–1057, 1997

Qureshi GA, Hansen S, Sodersten P: Offspring control of cerebrospinal fluid GABA concentrations in lactating rats. Neurosci Lett 75:85–88, 1987

Reul JM, Stec I, Soder M, et al: Chronic treatment of rats with the antidepressant amitriptyline attenuates the activity of the hypothalamic-pituitary adrenocortical system. Endocrinology 133:312–320, 1993

Rivas-Arancibia S, Vazquez-Pereyra F: Hormonal modulation of extinction responses induced by sexual steroid hormones in rats. Life Sci 54:363–367, 1994

Robel P, Baulieu EE: Neurosteroids: biosynthesis and function. Crit Rev Neurobiol 9:383–394, 1995

Rodier WI: Progesterone-estrogen interaction in the control of activity-wheel running in the female rat. Journal of Comparative and Physiological Psychology 74:365–373, 1971

Rodriguez-Sierra JF, Howard JL, Pollard GT, et al: Effect of ovarian hormones on conflict behavior. Psychoneuroendocrinology 9:293–300, 1984

Rodriguez-Sierra JF, Hagkey MT, Hendricks SE: Anxiolytic effects of progesterone are sexually dimorphic. Life Sci 38:1841–1845, 1986

Roozendaal BJ, McGaugh JL: Amygdaloid lesions differentially affect glucocorticoid-induced memory enhancement in an inhibitory avoidance task. Neurobiol Learn Mem 65:1–8, 1996

Rubinow D, Roy-Byrne PP: Premenstrual syndromes: overviews from a methodologic perspective. Am J Psychiatry 141:163–172, 1984

Rubinow D, Hoban M, Grover GN: Changes in plasma hormones across the menstrual cycle in patients with menstrually related mood disorder and in control subjects. Am J Obstet Gynecol 158:5–11, 1988

Rupprecht R, Hauser CA, Trapp T, et al: Neurosteroids: molecular mechanisms of action and psychopharmacologic significance. J Steroid Biochem Mol Biol 56:163–168, 1996

Schlein PA, Zarrow MX, Denenberg VH: The role of prolactin in the depressed or "buffered" adrenocorticosteroid response of the rat. J Endocrinol 62:93–99, 1974

Schmaltz LW, Isaacson RL: Effect of bilateral hippocampal destruction on the acquisition and extinction of an operant response. Physiol Behav 2:291–298, 1967

Schmidt PJ, Nieman LK, Danaceau MA, et al: Differential behavioral effects of gonadal steroids in women with and in those without premenstrual syndrome. N Engl J Med 338:209–216, 1998

Schumacher M, Coirini H, McEwen B: Regulation of high-affinity GABA$_A$ receptors in the dorsal hippocampus by estradiol and progesterone. Brain Res 487:178–183, 1989

Sheline YI, Wang PW, Gado MH, et al: Hippocampal atrophy in recurrent major depression. Proc Natl Acad Sci U S A 93:3908–3913, 1996

Simerly RB, Chang C, Muramatsu M, et al: Distribution of androgen and estrogen receptor mRNA-containing cells in the rat brain: an in situ hybridization study. J Comp Neurol 294:76–95, 1990

Singh M, Meyer EM, Millard WJ, et al: Ovarian steroid deprivation results in a reversible learning impairment and compromised cholinergic function in female Sprague-Dawley rats. Brain Res 644:305–312, 1994

Smith MS: Lactation alters neuropeptide-Y and proopiomelanocortin gene expression in the arcuate nucleus of the rat. Endocrinology 133:1258–1265, 1993

Smith SS: Estrogen administration increases neuronal responses to excitatory amino acids as a long term effect. Brain Res 503:354–357, 1989

Solomon BL, Fein HG, Smallridge RC: Usefulness of antimicrosomal antibody titers in the diagnosis and treatment of postpartum thyroiditis. J Fam Pract 36:177–182, 1993

Southwick S, Krystal J, Morgan C: Abnormal noradrenergic function in posttraumatic stress disorder. Arch Gen Psychiatry 50:266–274, 1993

Starkman M, Gebarski S, Berent S, et al: Hippocampal formation volume, memory dysfunction, and cortisol levels in patients with Cushing's syndrome. Biol Psychiatry 32:756–765, 1992

Steenbergen HL, Heinsbroek RPW, VanHaaren F, et al: Sex-dependent effects of inescapable shock administration on shuttlebox-escape performance and elevated plus-maze behavior. Physiol Behav 48:571–576, 1990

Steimer T, Driscoll P, Schulz PE: Brain metabolism of progesterone, coping behavior and emotional reactivity in male rats from two psychogenetically selected lines. J Neuroendocrinol 9:69–75, 1997

Suomi SJ: Primate separation models of affective disorders, in Neurobiology of Learning, Emotion and Affect. Edited by Madden J. New York, Raven, 1991, pp 195–214

Svec F, Yeakley J, Harrison RW: Progesterone enhances glucocorticoid dissociation from the AT-20 cell glucocorticoid receptor. Endocrinology 107:566–572, 1980

Terasawa E, Timiras PS: Electrical activity during the estrous cycle of the rat: cyclic changes in limbic structures. Endocrinology 83:207–216, 1967

Teyler TJ, Vardaris RM, Lewis D, et al: Gonadal steroids: effects on excitability of hippocampal pyramidal neurons. Science 209:1017–1019, 1980

Uht R, Anderson C, Webb P, et al: Transcriptional activities of estrogen and glucocorticoid receptors are functionally integrated at the AP-1 response element. Endocrinology 138:2900–2908, 1997

Uno H, Else JG, Suleman MA, et al: Hippocampal damage associated with prolonged and fatal stress in primates. J Neurosci 9:1705–1711, 1989

Walker CD, Lightman SL, Steele MK, et al: Suckling is a persistent stimulus to the adrenocortical system of the rat. Endocrinology 130:115–125, 1992

Warren SG, Humphries AG, Juraska JM, et al: LTP varies across the estrous cycle: enhanced synaptic plasticity in proestrus rats. Brain Res 703:26–30, 1995

Watts AG, Sanchez-Watts G: Region specific regulation of neuropeptide mRNA levels in neurones of the limbic forebrain by adrenal steroids. J Physiol (Lond) 484:721–736, 1995

Weiland N: Estradiol selectively regulates agonist binding sites on the N-methyl-D-aspartate receptor complex in the CA1 region of the hippocampus. Endocrinology 131:662–668, 1992a

Weiland N: Glutamic acid decarboxylase messenger ribonucleic acid is regulated by estradiol and progesterone in the hippocampus. Endocrinology 131:2697–2702, 1992b

Weisenfeld AR, Malatesta CZ, Whitman PB, et al: Psychophysiological response of breast- and bottle-feeding mothers to their infants' signals. Psychophysiology 22:79–86, 1985

Wiklund I, Karlberg J, Mattsson LA: Quality of life of postmenopausal women on a regimen of transdermal estradiol therapy: a double-blind, placebo-controlled study. Am J Obstet Gynecol 168:824–830, 1993

Willner P: Behavior models in psychopharmacology, in Behavioral Models in Psychopharmacology: Theoretical, Industrial and Clinical Perspectives. Edited by Willner P. Cambridge, UK, Cambridge University Press, 1991, pp 3–18

Wong M, Moss RL: Long-term and short-term electrophysiological effects of estrogen on the synaptic properties of hippocampal CA1 neurons. J Neurosci 12:3217–3225, 1992

Wong M, Thompson TL, Moss RL: Nongenomic actions of estrogen in the brain: physiological significance and cellular mechanisms. Crit Rev Neurobiol 10:189–203, 1996

Wood GE, Shors TJ: Stress facilitates classical conditioning in males, but impairs classical conditioning in females through activational effects of ovarian hormones. Proc Natl Acad Sci U S A 95:4066–4071, 1998

Woolley CS, McEwen BS: Estradiol mediates fluctuation in hippocampal synapse density during the estrous cycle in the adult rat. J Neurosci 12:2549–2554, 1992

Woolley CS, McEwen BS: Estradiol regulates hippocampal dendritic spine density via an N-methyl-D-aspartate receptor-dependent mechanism. J Neurosci 14:7680–7687, 1994

Yang J: Intrathecal administration of oxytocin induces analgesia in low back pain involving the endogenous opiate peptide system. Spine 19:867–871, 1994

Yehuda R, Boisoneau D, Lowy MT, et al: Dose-response changes in plasma cortisol and lymphocyte glucocorticoid receptors following dexamethasone administration in combat veterans with and without posttraumatic stress disorder. Arch Gen Psychiatry 52:583–593, 1995

Zhu Y, Yen P, Chin W, et al: Estrogen and thyroid hormone interaction on regulation of gene expression. Proc Natl Acad Sci U S A 93:12587–12592, 1996

Zweifel JE, O'Brien WH: A meta-analysis of the effect of hormone replacement therapy upon depressed mood. Psychoneuroendocrinology 22:189–212, 1997

Chapter 4

Hormone Replacement and Oral Contraceptive Therapy: Do They Induce or Treat Mood Symptoms?

Kimberly A. Yonkers, M.D., and
Karen D. Bradshaw, M.D.

It is commonly believed that exogenous progestins can precipitate mood disorders, such as major or minor depressive disorders (Backstrom 1995; Studd et al. 1977). On the other hand, some researchers and clinicians advocate the use of estrogens (Klaiber et al. 1996; Studd and Smith 1994) or progesterone (Dalton 1971) to treat mood disturbances or disorders. Progestins and estrogens are commonly used either for contraception or to treat postmenopausal symptoms and to decrease the risks of long-term hypogonadal complications (osteoporosis, cerebrovascular and cardiovascular disease). In the United States, an estimated 10 million postmenopausal women and 15 million reproductive-aged women are prescribed these hormones (Lobo 1994; personal communication, Ortho Pharmaceutical Corporation, 1996). Given the high likelihood that a woman will receive a prescription for exogenous gonadal hormones at some time during her life, there is a need to critically evaluate the risks and benefits associated with their use. For psychiatrists in particular, this means becoming aware of data regarding the contribution of these hormones toward inducing mood symptoms as well as toward providing any psychiatric benefits. In this chapter we review existing data on the psychiatric effects of exogenous estrogens and progestins used in oral contraceptive and hormone replacement regimens.

This review has been informed by other work published by our group (Yonkers and Bradshaw, in press).

A MEDLINE search for publications between 1966 and 1998 was conducted using the following keywords: hormones, estrogen, progestin, progestogen, oral contraceptives, mood, depression, menopause, and premenstrual syndrome. In addition, bibliographies of database and review articles were examined. Because of the difficulty of extrapolating unbiased results from open investigations (i.e., nonrandomized, non-placebo-controlled studies), this review focuses primarily on placebo-controlled investigations, although the findings of case–control studies and open studies are noted where appropriate.

Exogenous Estrogens and Progestins

In young women, the major circulating estrogen is the steroid molecule 17 β-estradiol. The less potent estrogen estrone is also produced in significant amounts through both direct ovarian secretion and peripheral aromatization of ovarian- and adrenal-derived androstenedione. The amount of estradiol varies between 40 and 400 pg/mL during the normal menstrual cycle. Estradiol circulates, while bound, to sex hormone–binding globulin (SHBG), which is produced by the liver. The quantity of SHBG produced is partially controlled by estrogen. A dramatic decline in the production of estradiol and estrone by the ovaries occurs after menopause. At the time of natural menopause, estradiol levels decrease to less than 40 pg/mL, while testosterone production declines by only 25%. The increased androgen-to-estrogen ratio leads to a reduction in SHBG, since androstenedione production declines slightly with age, and thus estrone, synthesized from androstenedione, becomes the major circulating estrogen after menopause.

Exogenous estrogens can be administered either orally or parenterally. Estrogens commonly used in oral contraceptives include ethinyl estradiol and mestranol. Ethinyl estradiol is synthesized by adding an ethinyl group at the 17th carbon position of the estradiol molecule, whereas mestranol is produced by adding a 3-methyl ether group to the ethinyl estradiol molecule; it is converted to ethinyl estradiol in vivo. Currently prescribed low-dose oral contraceptives contain ethinyl estradiol in doses of 20, 30, or 35 μg; these dosage ranges are three to four times more potent than those used in hormone replacement therapy (HRT) regimens. Higher-dose oral contraceptives containing 75–100 μg of ethinyl estradiol or mestranol are no longer available.

The most frequently used estrogens for HRT are conjugated equine estrogens, a combination of estrone (50%), equilin (23%), 17 α-dihydroequilin (13%), and various other estrogens extracted from the urine of pregnant mares (Lyman and Johnson 1982). These preparations have been available for more than 50 years, and thus, most of the data regarding the safety and efficacy of postmenopausal estrogen therapy have been gathered from women taking conjugated estrogens. Several other estrogen preparations have been developed, including piperazine estrone sulfate and micronized 17 β-estradiol, and data are accumulating regarding their comparable effectiveness. At present, there are no major differences in risks or side effects of any particular preparation.

Although transdermal 17 β-estradiol patches have also been found to be effective for HRT, there are several potential drawbacks associated with parenteral administration. It is uncertain whether similar reductions in cardio- and cerebrovascular risk occur with the transdermal estrogen as with oral preparations, because transdermally administered estrogen avoids the "first pass" through the liver and hence has less effect on low- and high-density lipids (Stanczyk et al. 1988). Also, patches are more expensive than most oral estrogens and cause skin irritation in about 30% of women. Transdermal 17 β-estradiol should be reserved for use in women who do not tolerate oral agents or who develop hypertriglyceridemia while taking an oral preparation. As will be discussed later in this chapter, transdermal 17 β-estradiol patches may also have a greater effect on mood than do synthetic formulations of estrogen. Table 4–1 lists standard dosages of commonly used estrogens.

Conjugated estrogens in cream form are also available, and rates of vaginal absorption are similar to those for oral absorption (Dickerson et al. 1979). Estrogen gels, implants, and injections

Table 4–1. Standard dosages of commonly used estrogens and progestins

Estrogens	Dosage range
Oral	
Conjugated estrogens	0.625–1.25 mg/day
Ethinyl estradiol	0.025–0.035 mg/day
Piperazine estrone sulfate	1.0 mg/day
Micronized 17 β-estradiol	0.5–2.0 mg/day
Mestranol	0.05 mg/day
Parenteral	
Transdermal estradiol	0.05–1.0 mg patch once or twice weekly
Vaginal conjugated estrogens	0.2–0.625 mg, 2–7 times weekly
Vaginal 17 β-estradiol	1.0 mg, 1–3 times weekly

Progestins	Dosage range
Oral	
Medroxyprogesterone acetate	2.5–5.0 mg/day or 10 mg 10–14 days per month
Norethindrone acetate	1–5 mg/day
Norgestrel	0.15 mg/day
Micronized progesterone	100–300 mg/day

Source. Reproduced with permission from Steiner M, Yonkers KA, Eriksson E: *Depression in Women.* London, Martin Dunitz Ltd., 1998.

are available but are rarely used because of their erratic absorption and the wide variations in blood levels they produce. The so-called natural estrogens (catecholestrogens) are available in health-food markets in the form of soy estrogens or yam extracts. Because neither the exact chemical nature of these products nor the appropriate dosing regimens are known, they should not be used for the treatment of postmenopausal symptoms.

Progesterone is a 21-carbon steroid that is synthesized from pregnenolone in the corpus luteum of ovulatory, reproductive-aged women. It is released in a manner best characterized as "pulsatile," with levels ranging from 5 to 50 mg/mL between the day of ovulation and the next menstrual period. Levels of progesterone peak in the midluteal phase of the cycle, around day 21 of a 28-day cycle. Low levels of progesterone are found during the follicular phase in ovulatory, anovulatory, and postmenopausal women.

Exogenous progesterone can be administered orally but has low bioavailability because it is poorly absorbed from the intestine. Two approaches have been used to synthesize orally active compounds. One strategy is to micronize the preparation. Products prepared in this fashion have been used in Europe for years and are now starting to be widely available in the United States. Progesterone has also been modified at the 17th carbon and the 6th carbon of the molecule to make the potent oral progestins medroxyprogesterone acetate and megestrol acetate. Another approach to synthesizing an orally active progestin for oral contraceptives is to modify the C-19 steroid testosterone. With removal of the 18th carbon and addition of an ethinyl group at the 17th carbon, testosterone is converted to norethindrone, norethindrone acetate, and norgestrel (Whitehead et al. 1990). As outlined in Table 4–1, progestins are available in several different formulations. The most frequently prescribed progestin for postmenopausal women is oral medroxyprogesterone acetate. However, as with estrogen preparations, no single progestin is clearly superior to any other. If a woman has significant side effects with one progestin preparation or dosage, a lower dosage or a different progestin formulation is recommended.

Effects of Estrogen and Progesterone on the Serotonergic System

Estrogen has a number of effects on neurotransmitter systems; these effects have been described in detail in other reports (Halbreich 1997; Halbreich and Lumley 1993; Steiner et al. 1997). Because of the possible association between serotonin and mood disorders, the relationship between estrogen and the serotonergic (5-hydroxytryptamine [5-HT]) system is of particular interest. More is known about estrogen's effects in the rat brain than in the human brain. In rats, estrogen treatment has been shown to decrease 5-HT_1 receptor density (Biegon et al. 1983) and to increase 5-HT_2 receptor density in the frontal cortex (Biegon et al. 1983; Fischette et al. 1983; Sumner and Fink 1995), as well as in the nucleus accumbens, cingulate cortex, and olfactory cortex (Fink et al. 1996; Sumner and Fink 1995). In the raphe, estrogen increases serotonin content by stimulating messenger RNA (mRNA) production of the serotonin-synthesizing enzyme tryptophan hydroxylase (Pecins-Thompson et al. 1996). Estrogen also inhibits monoamine oxidase activity (Jones and Naftolin 1990) and decreases the turnover of 5-HT (Shimizu and Bray 1993) in rodents. Less is known about the effects of estrogen in the central nervous system (CNS) of humans, although some information is available from models that putatively mimic the CNS. Estrogen increases platelet 5-HT$_2$ binding and is associated with increased binding in the platelet serotonin transporter (Rojansky et al. 1991). Finally, endogenous and exogenous estrogens increase the prolactin response to serotonin agonists (Halbreich et al. 1995; O'Keane et al. 1991). Recent evidence suggests that estrogen has activational effects. As reviewed by Smith (1994), estrogen increases locomotor activity and enhances the activity of excitatory amino acids in the CNS of rodents. The excitatory properties of estrogen may be responsible for its cognition-enhancing effects and may also relate to its mood-lifting effects (Kampen and Sherwin 1994; Phillips and Sherwin 1992; Sherwin 1994). Some of the properties of estrogen demonstrated in humans and animals are similar to those found in antidepressant agents, thus strengthening the proposition that estrogens may have mood-elevating properties.

In animal systems, the biological effects of an endogenous compound are often counterbalanced by the properties of other compounds. Such a balance can be seen with estrogen and progesterone. Whereas estrogen increases the receptor expression of many compounds, including itself, progesterone reverses the estrogen-induced receptor expression in selected areas of the brain. In short, this means that progesterone appears to temper the effects of estrogen (Pecins-Thompson et al. 1996; Smith 1994). This characteristic of progesterone is mediated both through its binding to nuclear receptors that influence RNA synthesis and through its nongenomic, membrane receptor–binding properties. The nongenomic activity occurs through the alpha-ring–reduced metabolites of progesterone, such as allopregnanolone, which bind to a specific site on the gamma-aminobutyric acid (GABA)–benzodiazepine receptor and increase the duration of channel opening (Mahesh et al. 1996; Majewska et al. 1986; Smith 1994). This activity is similar to that of barbiturates, which bind at a different site on the receptor complex and cause sedation (Smith 1994). In rat models of anxiety, selected progesterone metabolites decrease behavior associated with anxiety (Bitran et al. 1993). In humans, administration of progesterone can cause an increase in allopregnanolone levels that is associated with higher levels of fatigue (Freeman et al. 1993). Progesterone, like estrogen, decreases 5-HT$_1$ receptor density and increases 5-HT$_2$ receptor density in the frontal cortex (Biegon et al. 1983), but this effect is less pronounced with progesterone than with estrogen. Like estrogen, progesterone increases serotonin turnover in the brain (Gereau et al. 1993) and increases serotonin content in the raphe, although, again, to a lesser extent than does estrogen (Pecins-Thompson et al. 1996). In sum, while progesterone and its metabolites exert modulatory effects on estrogen, progesterone alone has important properties that are sometimes similar to those of estrogen.

Estrogen in the Treatment of Menopausal Mood Disorders

There is no perfect definition of perimenopause, although clinicians usually consider a woman perimenopausal if her menses are irregular and her day 4 follicular-stimulating hormone level is above 40 pg/mL. Menopause is defined as the last menstrual period. Most cross-sectional and longitudinal studies conducted in community settings have not shown an increase in mood disorders during the postmenopausal period (Ballinger 1975; Bungay et al. 1980; Hallstrom and Samuelsson 1985; Hunter et al. 1986; Kaufert et al. 1992; Matthews 1992; McKinlay et al. 1987) (also see Ballinger 1990 for a review). However, several community studies have found a slight increase in mood symptoms and milder mood disorders during the immediate premenopausal period (Ballinger 1975; Bungay et al. 1980; Hunter et al. 1986) and in women who undergo surgical menopause (McKinlay et al. 1987). A number of authors have found that the impact of the psychosocial events occurring during these years of a woman's life is as great as or greater than the impact of the biological changes underlying menopause in determining whether a menopausal woman will develop mood symptoms (Ballinger 1975; Bungay et al. 1980; Hallstrom and Samuelsson 1985; Matthews 1992; McKinlay et al. 1987). Despite the meager epidemiological support for a menopausal mood syndrome, many women in clinical samples endorse problems with mood during the perimenopausal or postmenopausal period. On the whole, approximately 35% of women will seek medical treatment for a variety of symptoms associated with menopause (Backstrom 1995). The most common complaints include hot flashes, muscle and joint pain, headaches, weight gain, decreased libido, fatigue, low mood, and irritability (Stuenkel 1989). Estrogen preparations have been used to treat menopausal symptoms, including the mood symptoms that often accompany physical symptoms.

Although estrogen is effective for the treatment of hot flashes, evidence for its therapeutic efficacy for mood symptoms is mixed. The lack of consensus regarding estrogen's effectiveness in treating menopause-associated mood disorders may, in large part, be due to heterogeneity in the design of the clinical trials that have tested its efficacy. Relevant methodological issues are as follows: 1) the enrollment of women who were at various menopausal stages, including perimenopause, nonsurgical postmenopause, and surgical menopause; 2) the inclusion of patients who varied in the severity of their mood disturbance; 3) the enrollment of women with concurrent psychiatric illness; 4) the utilization of different types of estrogens, both with and without a progestin; and 5) the use of different outcome measures, such as single-symptom measures, as well as validated and nonvalidated scales. In our review of estrogen's efficacy in menopause-related mood disturbances, we comment on these relevant factors. The reader is also referred to a recent quantitative review of the effect of estrogen on peri- and postmenopausal mood symptoms (Zweifel and O'Brien 1997). The review we present in the following sections considers the results from that meta-analysis, discusses additional variables, and includes more recent studies.

Placebo-Controlled Studies

Twenty-two placebo-controlled trials have tested estrogen's efficacy for depressive symptoms or for depressive disorders associated with menopause (Table 4–2). Of these, five studies (Coppen et al. 1977; Dennerstein and Burrows 1979; Ditkoff et al. 1991; George et al. 1973; Sherwin and Gelfand 1985) included only women who had undergone surgical menopause; eight studies included only women who had experienced natural menopause (Brincat et al. 1984; Campbell 1976; Derman et al. 1995; Fedor-Freybergh 1977; Furuhjelm et al. 1984; Klaiber et al. 1996; Saletu et al. 1995; Wiklund et al. 1993); five studies enrolled both peri- and postmenopausal women (Aylward et al. 1974; Coope 1981; Coope et al. 1975; Montgomery et al. 1987; Strickler et al. 1977); two studies limited participants to perimenopausal women (Schmidt et al. [submitted for publication]; Thomson and Oswald 1977); one study did not define the exact menopausal status of women included in the protocol (Gerdes et al. 1982); and one study included both surgically and naturally menopausal women (Paterson 1982).

Surgically Induced Menopause

In three (Dennerstein and Burrows 1979; Ditkoff et al. 1991; Sherwin and Gelfand 1985) of the five studies that enrolled surgically postmenopausal women, estrogen was superior to placebo in treating mood symptoms. A variety of estrogen preparations, including conjugated estrogens (Ditkoff et al. 1991), ethinyl estradiol (Dennerstein and Burrows 1979), and estradiol valerate (Sherwin and Gelfand 1985), were used in these investigations. The two studies that found estrogen and placebo to be equivalent in efficacy employed either estrogen sulfate (Coppen et al. 1977) or conjugated estrogen (George et al. 1973). Sample sizes in these studies varied, with the positive studies (i.e., those reporting beneficial effects for estrogen) tending to be slightly larger ($ns = 49, 36, 43$) than the negative studies ($ns = 28, 13$). These differences in sample size may be meaningful, because the larger studies had more power to show a difference in treatment conditions. The negative study by Coppen and colleagues (1977) was

Table 4-2. Studies evaluating the effects of estrogen in perimenopausal and postmenopausal women

Perimenopausal studies

Study	N	Duration	Design	Hormonal preparation	Posttreatment placebo	Posttreatment active	Comments
Aylward et al. 1974	55	1 month	Parallel	Piperazine estrone sulfate	HRSD change = (+) 20%	HRSD change = (−) 20%	Perimenopausal and postmenopausal women included; estrone significantly better than placebo; tryptophan levels increased with estrone treatment
Coope et al. 1975	30	1 month	Crossover	Conjugated estrogens; no progestin	24% with complete relief	29% with complete relief	Differences between conditions not found; hot flashes appeared with withdrawal of estrogen, unblinding investigators; 2 subjects on estrogen withdrew because of depression

Study	N	Duration	Design	Treatment			Comments
Coope 1981	55	4 months	Crossover	Piperazine estrone sulfate; no progestin	BDI change = (–) 11 points	BDI change = (–) 9 points	No significant treatment effect; mildly depressed subjects included; 2 subjects developed severe depression while taking estrogen
Montgomery et al. 1987	70	4 months	Parallel	2 active treatments: 1) estradiol; 2) estradiol and testosterone; 5 mg norethindrone for final week of month	Placebo change score = 11	Estradiol/ testosterone change score = 18	Treatment differences significant at 2 months but not at 4 months
Strickler et al. 1977	70	6 months	Crossover	Conjugated estrogens	Authors' scale = no difference between active treatment and placebo	Authors' scale = no difference between active treatment and placebo	3 were bipolar and 9 were depressed at some point before study; 9 taking psychotropics
Schmidt et al. (submitted for publication)	31	1 month	Parallel	Oral 17 β-estradiol	HRSD change = (–) 4 points	HRSD change = (–) 9.5 points	All patients had MDD; treatment effect on mood was independent of effect on somatic symptoms

(continued)

Table 4–2. Studies evaluating the effects of estrogen in perimenopausal and postmenopausal women *(continued)*

					Perimenopausal studies *(continued)*		
Study	N	Duration	Design	Hormonal preparation	Posttreatment placebo	Posttreatment active	Comments
Thomson and Oswald 1977	34	2 months	Crossover	Piperazine estrone sulfate	HRSD change = (–) 10.4 points	HRSD change = (–) 13.7 points	No significant difference between treatment conditions; estrogen did not decrease the number of awakenings in perimenopausal women

					Postmenopausal studies		
Study	N	Duration	Design	Hormonal preparation	Posttreatment placebo	Posttreatment active	Comments
Brincat et al. 1984	55	4 months	Parallel and single-blind	100 mg testosterone and estradiol implant 50 mg; 5 mg norethindrone last week of month	Change in depression item = (–) 0.1 point at 2 months and (–) 0.3 point at 4 months	Change in depression item = (–) 1.3 points at 2 months and (–) 1.1 points at 4 months	Return of symptoms after 4 months; estradiol and testosterone significantly better than placebo for all symptoms except "aches and pains"

Study	N	Duration	Design	Treatment			Comments
Campbell 1976	64	2 months	Crossover	Conjugated estrogens; no progestin	BDI change = (−) 4 points	BDI change = (−) 5 points	No significant treatment effect; no baseline assessment of psychopathology
Derman et al. 1995	82	4 months	Parallel	17 β-estradiol; sequential norethindrone acetate	BDI change = (−) 0.1 point	BDI change = (−) 2.0 points	The most profound change occurred in vasomotor symptoms, but mild mood symptoms improved with active treatment
Fedor-Freybergh 1977	50	3 months	Parallel	Oral estradiol; progestin added days 13–22	HRSD change = (+) 3 points	HRSD change = (−) 9 points	Estrogen significantly better than placebo; subjects with baseline psychopathology excluded
Furuhjelm et al. 1984 (3 groups stratified for severity at baseline)	48	2 months	Crossover	Oral estradiol and estriol; norethindrone during final week	Change scores: severe = 1.2; moderate = 1.1; minimal = 0.7 points	Change scores: severe = 5.5; moderate = 1.3; minimal = 1.9 points	Treatment effect for depression strongest in most symptomatic group

(continued)

Table 4–2. Studies evaluating the effects of estrogen in perimenopausal and postmenopausal women (*continued*)

| | | | | Postmenopausal studies (*continued*) | | |
Study	N	Duration	Design	Hormonal preparation	Posttreatment placebo	Posttreatment active	Comments
Klaiber et al. 1996	38	1 month	Parallel	Estropipate and placebo or estropipate and nor-ethindrone, placebo	HRSD change = (–) 8.8 points	HRSD change = (–) 7.7 points	Mood and anxiety slightly worsened in estropipate and placebo cycle (nonsignificant)
Saletu et al. 1995	64	3 months	Parallel	Transdermal estradiol; no progestin	HRSD change = (–) 10.3 points	HRSD change = (–) 9.6 points	All subjects met criteria for MDD; high non-specific response rate in placebo group
Wiklund et al. 1993	242	3 months	Parallel	Transdermal estradiol; no progestin	Psychological well-being change = (–) 6.5 points	Psychological well-being change = (–) 13.5 points	Significant improvement in several measures of psychological health, including depression; subjects with psychiatric illness excluded

Postsurgical menopause studies

Study	N	Duration	Design	Hormonal preparation	Posttreatment placebo	Posttreatment active	Comments
Coppen et al. 1977	28	6 months with follow-up;	Parallel	Piperazine estrone sulfate; no progestin	BDI change = (−) 4.5 points in matched group at 6 months	BDI change = (−) 5.6 points in matched group at 6 months	Groups differed significantly at baseline on BDI; response in matched groups not significantly different
	18	1 year with follow-up					
Dennerstein and Burrows 1979	49	3 months	Crossover	3 active treatments: 1) ethinyl estradiol; 2) levonorgestrel; 3) ethinyl estradiol and levonorgestrel	HRSD change = (+) 4.3 points	HRSD change = (+) 1.9 points ethinyl estradiol; (+) 3.4 points levonorgestrel; (+) 2.8 points combined	Excluded subjects with psychiatric illness; best response in subjects taking estrogen
Ditkoff et al. 1991	13	3 months	Parallel	Conjugated estrogens; no progestin	BDI change = (+) 2 points	BDI change = (−) 2 points	Included only "asymptomatic" subjects at baseline; significant difference between groups

(continued)

Table 4–2. Studies evaluating the effects of estrogen in perimenopausal and postmenopausal women (*continued*)

Study	N	Duration	Design	Hormonal preparation	Posttreatment placebo	Posttreatment active	Comments
Postsurgical menopause studies (*continued*)							
George et al. 1973	13	1 month	Crossover	Conjugated estrogens; no progestin	BDI change = (−) 13 points	BDI change = (−) 11 points	All subjects were started on active treatment and then switched to estrogen or placebo; no significant difference between treatment conditions
Sherwin and Gelfand 1985	43	3 months	Crossover	Estrogen or androgen or combination	MAACL change = (+) 3 points	MAACL change = (−) 3 points	Significant treatment difference; groups evaluated with MAACL at baseline
Paterson 1982	20	3 months	Crossover	Mestranol and norethindrone	Authors' scale: Group 1 = (−) 0.6 point; Group 2 = 0 points	Authors' scale: Group 1 = 0 points; Group 2 = (−) 0.3 point	Mood scores showed symptoms improved in the first 3 months, regardless of treatment condition

Other postmenopausal study

Study	N	Duration	Design	Hormonal preparation	Posttreatment placebo	Posttreatment active	Comments
Gerdes et al. 1982	38	5 months	Parallel	Conjugated estrogens; medroxyprogesterone days 16–21	Not enough information	Not enough information	Improvement in mood symptoms significantly greater in estrogen group vs. placebo group

Note. Authors' scale = scale developed by authors of study; BDI = Beck Depression Inventory (Beck et al. 1961); HRSD = Hamilton Rating Scale for Depression (Hamilton 1960); MAACL = Multiple Adjective Affect Checklist (Zuckerman and Lubin 1965); MDD = major depressive disorder.
Source. Reproduced with permission from Steiner M, Yonkers KA, Eriksson E: *Depression in Women.* London, Martin Dunitz Ltd., 1998.

also hampered by substantial heterogeneity in illness severity at baseline, which may have further obfuscated differences in treatment outcomes.

Several aspects of the studies reporting beneficial effects for estrogen deserve comment. One study reporting a benefit for estradiol valerate (Sherwin et al. 1985) compared this compound with testosterone enanthate, a combination of estradiol valerate and testosterone enanthate, and placebo. Women who were randomized to placebo were more likely to experience mood deterioration, whereas women assigned to hormonal treatment experienced improved mood. Mood was most elevated in the testosterone-only group, but this treatment also resulted in the highest increase in hostility scores.

A study conducted in a Hispanic-American population (Ditkoff et al. 1991) excluded women experiencing substantial mood or physical symptoms at baseline. Despite the minimal symptoms among women in this study, the group assigned to conjugated estrogens exhibited greater improvement in mood than did the group assigned to placebo.

The third study to show benefit for estrogen randomized women to one of four treatment cells: ethinyl estradiol alone, ethinyl estradiol in combination with levonorgestrel, levonorgestrel alone, and placebo (Dennerstein and Burrows 1979). At baseline, one woman was moderately to severely depressed, eight women were moderately depressed, and the remaining women were not depressed. Women who received estrogen alone fared best, while the placebo group had the worst outcome. The baseline severity of mood disturbance did not influence treatment response.

Naturally Occurring Menopause

Eight studies included women who were naturally postmenopausal (Brincat et al. 1984; Campbell 1976; Derman et al. 1995; Fedor-Freybergh 1977; Furuhjelm et al. 1984; Klaiber et al. 1996; Saletu et al. 1995; Wiklund et al. 1993), and one included a mixed group of surgical and naturally postmenopausal women (Paterson 1982). In five of these nine studies (Brincat et al. 1984; Derman et al. 1995; Fedor-Freybergh 1977; Furuhjelm et al. 1984; Wiklund et al. 1993), estrogen treatment was more palliative for mood symptoms than was placebo. Medications used in these five positive studies included parenteral and oral estradiol. In one study, parenterally administered 17 β-estradiol with testosterone was significantly superior to placebo in alleviating somatic and psychological symptoms (Brincat et al. 1984). In another investigation, oral estradiol with sequential norethindrone improved mood symptoms, although the improvement in mood was not as great as the improvement in hot flashes (Derman et al. 1995).

The findings described above are reinforced by the results of a large study ($n = 223$) that evaluated 50 μg transdermal 17 β-estradiol in a group of mildly symptomatic women (Wiklund et al. 1993). The 50 μg 17 β-estradiol was significantly more beneficial than placebo in improving psychological well-being and alleviating anxiety and depression, as well as in relieving vasomotor symptoms.

Oral micronized estrogen was used in a study (Furuhjelm et al. 1984) that stratified women at baseline into those experiencing mild, moderate, or severe "depression" or "mental distress." Although all three groups experienced improvement in mental distress, only the severely depressed group showed greater improvement with estrogen than with placebo. Notably, women in this group continued to experience moderately severe symptoms after treatment.

Results from a small ($n = 20$) crossover study of naturally and surgically menopausal women that used the synthetic estrogen mestranol followed by the addition of norethindrone found that mestranol was superior to placebo for night sweats and flushing but not for mood symptoms (Paterson 1982).

A trial that specifically evaluated postmenopausal women ($n = 69$) with major depressive disorder (MDD) found no difference between 50 μg transdermal 17 β-estradiol and placebo (Saletu et al. 1995). The nonspecific (placebo) response rate was very high in this study, with 63% of the 17 β-estradiol group and 65% of the placebo group experiencing symptom improvement. A high nonspecific response rate was also found in an earlier study of 64 minimally symptomatic women receiving either conjugated estrogen or placebo (Campbell 1976; Campbell and Whitehead

1977). The null finding in these two studies resulted not from any finding of low efficacy for estrogen but rather from a high rate of response to placebo. Nonetheless, such high nonspecific response rates make it difficult to show a benefit for active drug treatment.

Perimenopause

A total of seven studies evaluated estrogen treatment in perimenopausal women. Two of the studies enrolled perimenopausal women only (Schmidt et al. [submitted for publication]; Thomson and Oswald 1977), and the other five studies enrolled both perimenopausal and postmenopausal women (Aylward et al. 1974; Coope 1981; Coope et al. 1975; Montgomery et al. 1987; Strickler et al. 1977).

Three of the seven studies showed a favorable response to estrogen (Aylward et al. 1974; Montgomery et al. 1987; Schmidt et al. [submitted for publication]). The earliest of these positive studies was an investigation using estrone sulfate; as mood improved, free tryptophan levels increased (Aylward et al. 1974). In the second study, 17 β-estradiol either alone or in conjunction with testosterone was compared with placebo in peri- and postmenopausal women (Montgomery et al. 1987). Women in this study were quite symptomatic; baseline scores in 86% of the subjects were consistent with psychiatric illness. Although improvement occurred in both peri- and postmenopausal women in all treatment cells, the change with active treatment was greater in the perimenopausal group than in the postmenopausal group and after 2 months was significantly greater than the change that occurred with placebo. After 4 months, however, the benefit with hormonal therapy was lost, a result that may have been due to either diminished hormonal levels (from the implants) or continued improvement in the placebo-treated group.

Finally, Schmidt and colleagues (submitted for publication) investigated the efficacy of oral estradiol versus placebo in 31 perimenopausal women with MDD. Hamilton Rating Scale for Depression (Hamilton 1960) scores showed a significantly greater decrease in the women receiving active treatment than in those receiving placebo. Furthermore, the decrease in mood symptoms occurred regardless of whether hot flashes remitted, suggesting that the mood improvement was not simply the result of an amelioration of physical symptoms.

The four studies that failed to demonstrate estrogen's superior effectiveness in comparison with placebo used either conjugated equine estrogen (two studies) (Coope et al. 1975; Strickler et al. 1977) or estrone sulfate (two studies) (Coope 1981; Thomson and Oswald 1977). Two of these trials (Coope 1981; Strickler et al. 1977) are difficult to interpret because some of the women had concurrent psychiatric illnesses and were allowed to continue psychotropic medication during the studies. It is probable that the underlying psychopathology in these women constituted a greater contribution to their mood symptoms than did the effect of menopause. The previously mentioned issue of high nonspecific response is germane to the remaining negative perimenopause studies (Coope et al. 1975; Thomson and Oswald 1977). This reinforces the need to include a placebo control when evaluating the efficacy of estrogen treatment.

Non-Placebo-Controlled Studies

Several non-placebo-controlled studies of estrogen in the treatment of menopausal mood disorders merit mention. Gerdes and colleagues (1982) administered HRT consisting of daily conjugated estrogen and 14 days of medroxyprogesterone versus the antihypertensive drug clonidine to 38 women. These two groups were compared with a third, no-treatment, group. The group receiving estrogen and medroxyprogesterone showed the greatest benefit, which included improvement on a variety of personality measures and on a self-report mood measure.

The findings of a longitudinal study by Maoz and Durst (1980) suggested that estrogen treatment of longer duration may have a greater impact on mood. In this study, women who remained on estrogen for 1 year had improved mood and sexual functioning compared with women who discontinued treatment. Of course, there could have been other factors that contributed to estrogen discontinuation, such as mood disorders causing apathy and decreased motivation.

In a large cross-sectional epidemiological study ($n = 1,200$) of women over 50 years of age, depressive symptoms occurred most often in women between the ages of 50 and 60 but were lower in the over-60 age group (Palinkas and Barrett-Connor 1992). The authors suggested that symptomatic women sought treatment and hence had higher initial rates during the 50- to 60-year interval. However, over time and with hormonal treatment, these women may have improved, thus explaining the more favorable scores in the HRT-treated women older than 60 years.

Finally, in an open study of postmenopausal women by de Lignieres and Vincens (1982), the mood- and anxiety-alleviating effects of exogenous estrogen and progesterone were investigated. Estrogen was well tolerated at lower doses but produced anxiety at higher doses. The longer the women remained on estrogen, the more their anxiety increased. These investigators reported that the anxiety-producing effect of estrogen were tempered by progesterone administration. This finding reinforces the abovementioned principle regarding the balance that exists between these two hormones—that is, progesterone may mitigate the activating effects of estrogen.

Estrogen in the Treatment of Nonmenopausal Mood Disorders

Estrogen has been investigated as a treatment for nonmenopausal mood disorders in nine studies: two monotherapy trials (Klaiber et al. 1979; Michael et al. 1970) and four adjunct therapy trials (Prange et al. 1977; Schneider et al. 1997, 1998; Shapira et al. 1985) in women with MDD, one trial in women with postpartum MDD (Gregoire et al. 1996), and three trials in women with premenstrual syndrome (PMS) (Dhar and Murphy 1991; Magos et al. 1986; Watson et al. 1989).

Estrogen as monotherapy for severe nonmenopausal MDD was tested in an early study of 40 female inpatients (Klaiber et al. 1979). This trial used extremely high doses of conjugated estrogen (5 mg/day increased to a maximum dosage of 25 mg/day). Even though the 23 women receiving estrogen improved significantly more than the women in the placebo group, posttreatment depression scores in the estrogen group remained moderate to severe, suggesting that this intervention is not satisfactory by itself. This study has not been replicated in a similar patient group.

Several trials have evaluated estrogen as an adjunct therapy for MDD. An early study (Prange et al. 1977) tested the benefit of adding estrogen to a tricyclic antidepressant (TCA), but found that even when positive effects of estrogen were initially seen, they were no longer apparent after 2 weeks. The high-dose estrogen plus TCA patients ultimately fared less well than the low-dose estrogen plus TCA patients or the TCA-only patients. Similarly negative results were reported for a small study (Shapira et al. 1985) of 11 women who were treated with the TCA imipramine and then randomized to adjunctive conjugated estrogen (at doses of up to 3.75 mg/day) or placebo. On the other hand, a secondary analysis from a large clinical trial investigated the effect of HRT on antidepressant response in older women (Schneider et al. 1997). Slightly greater improvement was found in the fluoxetine-treated women receiving HRT compared with the fluoxetine-treated women not receiving HRT. However, the women receiving HRT without fluoxetine did less well than the women receiving neither HRT nor fluoxetine, a finding that makes the results of this study difficult to interpret. Finally, a recent database reanalysis of elderly women treated with the SSRI sertraline either with or without concomitant HRT found that exogenous hormone use enhanced the likelihood of antidepressant response (Schneider et al. 1998).

An early investigation evaluated the effects of estrogen versus placebo on personality and functional impairment in older women (ages 60–91 years) (Michael et al. 1970). The Hospital Adjustment Scale (HAS; McReynolds 1968) was used to measure changes in interpersonal relationships and functioning, self-care, social responsibilities, and activities. Compared with women assigned to placebo, women assigned to estrogen improved on all measures and sustained better functioning over time. However, it was not clear whether the benefit seen with estrogen was secondary to estrogen's mood-elevating properties or attributable to its salutory effects on cognitive functioning (Barrett-Connor and Kritz-Silverstein 1993; Halbreich 1997).

There is some evidence that estrogen may have a role in the treatment of postpartum MDD. Sixty-four women with postpartum MDD were treated with either transdermal 17 β-estradiol or placebo for 6 months (Gregoire et al. 1996). The 17 β-estradiol–treated group had a better response, both statistically and clinically, compared with the placebo group. However, one-half of the women in this trial were also taking standard antidepressants, so it is not known whether 17 β-estradiol was effective as an adjunctive treatment or as monotherapy.

Estrogen has been used to treat the mood symptoms seen with PMS in three trials. Two of these studies (Magos et al. 1986; Watson et al. 1989) compared parenteral 17 β-estradiol with placebo, while the third study used conjugated estrogens (Dhar and Murphy 1991). 17 β-Estradiol was more effective than placebo for premenstrual dysphoria (Magos et al. 1986; Watson et al. 1989), but conjugated estrogens demonstrated no such benefit (Dhar and Murphy (1991). The study employing conjugated estrogens included only 11 women, and thus the failure to find a significant difference may be attributable to a lack of power.

Summary of Studies
Using Estrogen

The quantitative review by Zweifel and O'Brien (1997) concluded that estrogen treatment of menopausal women had a moderate to large beneficial effect on mood. The effect size was larger among perimenopausal than among postmenopausal women. It was also larger for natural versus surgically induced menopause. Finally, treatment for longer than 8 months was associated with the greatest improvement. In the qualitative review presented above, our conclusions were similar, with the exception that the benefits of estrogen treatment appeared to be more consistent in surgically menopausal women than in naturally menopausal women. However, most women included in the surgically postmenopausal group were mildly symptomatic, making it difficult to reach conclusions regarding the role of estrogen in surgically postmenopausal women with severe depressive symptoms (such as those seen in MDD).

Studies using estrogen as monotherapy for MDD have reported mixed results. Saletu and co-workers (1995) found estrogen and placebo equivalent in ameliorating postmenopausal MDD. Similarly, earlier studies by Prange et al. (1977) and Shapira et al. (1985) found no benefit of estrogen augmentation in MDD. Klaiber and colleagues (1979) did find statistical benefit for very high doses of estrogen in nonreproductive-related MDD, but these results were clinically insignificant. The database reanalyses by Schneider and co-workers (1997, 1998) are provocative but not definitive, since other factors leading to HRT use could have benefited mood in these subjects (e.g., greater optimism, better overall self-care). On the other hand, for the clearly reproductive-related mood disorders (PMS, perimenopausal MDD, and postpartum MDD), estrogen is clinically and statistically superior to placebo. It is likely that estrogen's role is stronger in these conditions.

Our review included several negative studies not included in the quantitative meta-analysis by Zweifel and O'Brien (1997) and was limited to placebo-controlled studies. A meta-analysis can estimate overall effect sizes summed from a number of studies. However, the validity of the meta-analysis is constrained by the fact that studies have substantial differences in design, outcome, and inclusion criteria (e.g., some studies enrolled women with current psychiatric illness and heterogeneous symptom severity). Also, given the high nonspecific response rate seen in several studies, the inclusion of noncontrolled estrogen studies in the meta-analysis may have biased the results favorably toward estrogen.

None of the aforementioned studies compared one estrogen preparation with another. However, the trials that most reliably detected a drug–placebo difference employed parenteral or transdermal 17 β-estradiol. Only one of six studies that used 17 β-estradiol found no difference between drug and placebo (Saletu et al. 1995), whereas a null result was found in 9 of 12 studies that used an estrogen compound composed predominantly of estrone. Importantly, 17 β-estradiol is a more biologically active estrogen than is estrone; estrone has only one-tenth of 17 β-estradiol's biological activity. Our review suggests the possibility that 17 β-estradiol is more effective than estrone in ameliorating mood symptoms associated with peri- or postmenopause.

Progestins in the Treatment of Menopausal Mood Disorders

Several authors have suggested that the palliative effects of estrogen on peri- and postmenopausal mood disorders are reversed by the addition of a progestational agent (Backstrom 1995; Studd and Smith 1994). Seven studies have investigated the effects of progestin on menopausal mood symptoms (Bullock et al. 1975; Kirkham et al. 1991; Klaiber et al. 1996; Magos et al. 1986; Morrison et al. 1980; Prior et al. 1994; Sherwin 1991); of these seven, four added progestin or placebo to ongoing estrogen therapy (Kirkham et al. 1991; Klaiber et al. 1996; Magos et al. 1986; Sherwin 1991) and three used only progestin or placebo (Bullock et al. 1975; Morrison et al. 1980; Prior et al. 1994) (Table 4–3).

An early open study, reported in three published papers (Backstrom 1995; Hammarback et al. 1985; Holst et al. 1989), showed a mild reversal in mood improvement among women treated in an open study design with percutaneous estradiol when a progestin was added. Several double-blind, placebo-controlled studies followed these reports, but their findings were mixed. In a study of 58 postmenopausal women treated with percutaneous estradiol (Magos et al. 1986), either norethindrone at a dosage of 2.5 or 5.0 mg/day or placebo was added for 7 days. Daily ratings for concentration and negative affect were slightly but significantly worse in the group receiving estradiol plus norethindrone compared with the group receiving estradiol plus placebo. No placebo-only group was included for comparison.

Similarly, a trial by Sherwin (1991) randomized 48 women to four groups: high-dose (1.25 mg/day) conjugated estrogens plus placebo, high-dose conjugated estrogens plus 5 mg/day medroxy-progesterone (days 15–25), low-dose (0.625 mg/day) conjugated estrogens plus placebo, and low-dose conjugated estrogens plus 5 mg/day of medroxyprogesterone (days 15–25). Although mood improved from baseline in all groups, the least improvement occurred in the medroxyprogesterone groups. What is puzzling is

Table 4–3. Studies evaluating the mood effects of progestins in perimenopausal and postmenopausal women

Study	N	Duration	Design	Hormonal preparation	Posttreatment placebo	Posttreatment active	Comments
Bullock et al. 1975	69	6 months	Parallel	Depot medroxy-progesterone	10% with side effect of depressed mood	10% with side effect of depressed mood	No difference between groups in onset of depression
Kirkham et al. 1991	48 (surgical postmenopausal)	1 month	Crossover	Transdermal estrogen days 1–25; medroxyprogesterone vs. placebo days 12–15	BDI: former-PMS group = 7.2 points; non-PMS group = 5.4 points	BDI: former-PMS group = 6.3 points; non-PMS group = 5.5 points	Half of subjects diagnosed with PMS; no difference in treatment condition for either former-PMS or non-PMS group
Klaiber et al. 1996	38	1 month	Parallel	Estropipate and placebo or estropipate and norethindrone	HRSD change = (−) 8.8 points	HRSD change = (−) 7.7 points	Mood and anxiety worsened in estropipate and placebo cycle (nonsignificant)

(continued)

Table 4–3. Studies evaluating the mood effects of progestogens in perimenopausal and postmenopausal women *(continued)*

Study	N	Duration	Design	Hormonal preparation	Posttreatment placebo	Posttreatment active	Comments
Magos et al. 1986	70 (surgical postmenopausal)	1 month	Parallel	Group 1: transdermal estradiol with 5 mg norethindrone vs. placebo ($n = 50$) Group 2: estradiol with 2.5 mg norethindrone vs. placebo ($n = 20$)	MDQ: Negative affect did not change with placebo in Group 1 or 2	MDQ: Negative affect changed 0.25 point with 5 mg and 0.05 point with 2.5 mg norethindrone	Somatic symptoms and negative affect worsened in Group 1; differences were very small
Prior et al. 1994	11 (postmenopausal)	2 months	Crossover	Medroxyprogesterone	Author daily diary: mood worsened 1 point	Author daily diary: mood improved 1 point	No significant worsening of somatic symptoms; no mood worsening with progestin; very small sample size

Study	N	Duration	Design	Treatment	Outcome	Outcome	Comments
Sherwin 1991	48	12 months	Parallel	0.625 mg conjugated estrogen and medroxyprogesterone or placebo; 1.25 mg conjugated estrogen and medroxyprogesterone	Daily rating calendar: addition of placebo increased positive mood score in 3rd week	Daily rating calendar: addition of progestin decreased positive mood score in 3rd week	Despite intermittent administration of progestin, scores differed between groups with added progestin and placebo
Morrison et al. 1980	48	3 months	Parallel	Depot medroxyprogesterone	Onset of depression = 25% in placebo group	Onset of depression = 6% in medroxyprogesterone group	Results are from side-effect data; well-being and somatic symptoms improved more with medroxyprogesterone

Note. Author daily diary = diary method developed by authors of study; BDI = Beck Depression Inventory (Beck et al. 1961); HRSD = Hamilton Rating Scale for Depression (Hamilton 1960); MDQ = Menstrual Distress Questionnaire (Moos 1968); PMS = premenstrual syndrome.
Source. Reproduced with permission from Steiner M, Yonkers KA, Eriksson E: *Depression in Women.* London, Martin Dunitz Ltd., 1998.

that this effect endured beyond the duration of progestin exposure. All groups had cyclical variation in mood throughout the month, with the greatest variation in the high-dose estrogen and placebo group.

Several investigators failed to find significant differences between placebo and progestin when these agents were added back to ongoing estrogen therapy (Kirkham et al. 1991; Klaiber et al. 1996). In a study of surgically menopausal women, mood changes after hormone treatment were compared in women who did versus those who did not have a history of PMS (Kirkham et al. 1991). Reversal of mood improvement after progestin treatment was no more likely to occur in women with a history of PMS than in women without such a history; neither group experienced a difference in mood symptoms with progestin compared with placebo add-back. Similar results were reported in another study that failed to find a significant difference in mood after the addition of progestin or placebo to estrone piperazine therapy (Klaiber et al. 1996).

Progestins were used as monotherapy for menopausal symptoms in three studies that provided limited information on the subjects' mood symptoms. The first of these, a small ($n = 11$), placebo-controlled crossover trial (Prior et al. 1994), investigated the mood-changing effects of medroxyprogesterone taken over the course of 2 months. Mood scores did not differ between the placebo and the progestin conditions. In the second study (Bullock et al. 1975), conducted in a heterogeneous group of surgically and naturally menopausal women, depot medroxyprogesterone ($n = 57$) or placebo ($n = 12$) was given for 6 months to control menopausal symptoms. Hot flashes diminished with the active treatment, and the potential side effect of transient depression was no more likely to occur in the active-treatment group than in the placebo group. Depot medroxyprogesterone was also investigated in the third study (Morrison et al. 1980), which collected side-effect information from 48 women taking the drug for menopausal symptoms. Once again, the rate of depressive symptoms was no higher in the medroxyprogesterone-treated women than in the placebo-treated women.

In sum, several but not all of these trials showed diminished mood-elevating effects when a progestin was added to estrogen treatment. In the studies that found a progestin effect, the magnitude of change in mood was not large. In addition, some postmenopausal women appear to experience monthly fluctuations in mood, even if they are taking only the estrogen component of HRT; for women receiving both estrogen and progestin, clinicians and patients may misattribute mood symptoms to the progestin. Finally, the most problematic mood changes in one placebo-controlled study (Sherwin 1991) occurred with high-dose versus low-dose estrogen, regardless of whether a progestin was also administered.

The effects of adding a progestin to ongoing estrogen treatment were probed in the meta-analysis by Zweifel and O'Brien (1997), with results supportive of our own conclusions. Although estrogen in combination with a progestin still improved mood, the effect was less pronounced than that found with estrogen alone.

Oral Contraceptives and Mood

Oral contraceptives (OCs) are commonly thought to contribute to mood disorders, and, indeed, this warning is included in the package insert of many OCs. Unfortunately, most of the evidence supporting this contention is based on anecdote and a few cross-sectional, uncontrolled studies rather than on either longitudinal or placebo-controlled trials. This literature was last reviewed in the early 1980s (Slap 1981). Since that time, two notable additional studies have been published (Graham and Sherwin 1993; Graham et al. 1995), yielding a total of four placebo-controlled studies bearing on this question (Table 4–4). One of these studies evaluated mood in women with PMS (Graham and Sherwin 1993) and thus might not be applicable to women without this diagnosis.

The first controlled study of OC effects on mood compared placebo with four different hormone preparations: a high-dose estrogen–sequential progestin pill, a high-dose estrogen–progestin combination pill, a low-dose estrogen–progestin combination pill, and a progestin-only pill (Goldzieher et al. 1971a, 1971b).

Table 4-4. Placebo-controlled studies evaluating the effects of oral contraceptives (OCs) on mood and other selected symptoms

Study	N	Disorder	Duration	Design	Hormonal preparation	Post-treatment placebo	Post-treatment active	Comments
Goldzieher et al. 1971a, 1971b	398	Not ill	1 month	Cross-over	Sequential ethinyl estradiol 0.1 mg/dimethisterone 25 mg	Author scale: 0.42 point	Author scale: 0.47 point	Symptoms varied slightly cycle by cycle; no significant differences in rates of depressive symptoms; higher score means more symptoms. Somewhat higher rate of nervousness in high-estrogen preparations. The crossover part of the study showed that subjects who had symptoms while taking placebo continued to have symptoms when they were crossed over to active treatment. The difference between conditions was very small; subjects taking "estrogen dominant" compound fared the least well overall.
					Mestranol 0.1 mg/ethynodiol diacetate 1 mg	0.42 point	0.62 point	
					Mestranol 0.5 mg/norethindrone 1 mg	0.42 point	0.49 point	
					Chlormadinone 0.5 mg daily and continuously	0.42 point	0.33 point	

Study	N	Population	Duration	Design	Drug	Author scale:	Author scale:	Comments
Cullberg 1972	240	Not ill	—	—	Norgestrel 1.0 mg/ ethinyl estradiol 0.05 mg	Mean score = (+) 0.2 point	Mean score = (+) 0 points	Higher score means more depression.
					Norgestrel 0.5 mg/ ethinyl estradiol 0.05 mg	Mean score = (+) 0.2 point	Mean score = (+) 0 points	
					Norgestrel 0.06 mg/ ethinyl estradiol 0.05 mg	Mean score = (+) 0.2 point	Mean score = (−) 0.4 point	
Graham and Sherwin 1993	82	PMS	3 months	Parallel	Ethinyl estradiol 0.035 mg and norethindrone 0.25 mg	N/A	N/A	Group with depressive symptoms at baseline did significantly better while taking OCs than while taking placebo.

(continued)

Table 4–4. Placebo-controlled studies evaluating the effects of oral contraceptives (OCs) on mood and other selected symptoms *(continued)*

Study	N	Disorder	Duration	Design	Hormonal preparation	Post-treatment placebo	Post-treatment active	Comments
Graham et al. 1995	150	Not ill	4 months	Parallel	Ethinyl estradiol 0.03 mg and levonorgestrel 0.15 mg		BDI change: Manila site = (+) 0.1 point; Edinburgh site = (+) 0.1 point	Study conducted in Manila, Philippines, and Edinburgh, Scotland. Mood was evaluated with daily ratings; increase in ratings indicates worse mood. Greatest reduction occurred in mood symptom scores.
					Levonorgestrel 0.03 mg	BDI change: Manila site = (+) 0.1 point; Edinburgh site = (+) 0.1 point	BDI change: Manila site = (−) 0.1 point; Edinburgh site = (−) 0.15 point	

Note. Author scale = scale developed by author(s) of study; BDI = Beck Depression Inventory (Beck et al. 1961); N/A = not applicable; PMS = premenstrual syndrome.
Source. Reproduced with permission from Steiner M, Yonkers KA, Eriksson E: *Depression in Women.* London, Martin Dunitz Ltd., 1998.

Women (n = 80 per cell) were treated for four cycles, after which women from some groups were crossed over to an alternative pill. During the first three cycles, the percentage of patients reporting depressed mood was approximately equal in all groups. Women were more likely to report nervousness than depression in all treatment groups, including the placebo group. An endorsement of anxious mood occurred slightly and nonsignificantly more often in the women given the high-dose estrogen–progestin combination pill. On average, women's reports of depressed mood gradually diminished over the 6 months of the study, essentially not supporting an overall deleterious effect for OCs on mood.

A similar strategy was employed in a second study that compared three different combination OC preparations and placebo (Cullberg 1972). Each group consisted of approximately 80 women who were treated with either placebo or norgestrel at a daily dose of 1.0 mg, 0.5 mg, or 0.06 mg combined with a fixed dose of ethinyl estradiol. This carefully designed study used several outcome measures, including an assessment of whether mood improved or deteriorated with treatment. Any mood changes were predominantly negative for all conditions. When the item "depressed mood" was evaluated, placebo-treated women experienced the least change (5%) compared with hormone-treated women (8% in the high-dose, 5% in the intermediate-dose, and 6% in the low-dose group), although the differences were not significant. The group that reported the largest degree of "negative mood change" was the low-dose estrogen–norgestrel group, and this difference was statistically significant. "Dysphoric" changes were somewhat higher in degree than "depressed mood" changes among all groups, and dysphoric changes were significantly more likely to be reported in the hormone groups than in the placebo group.

Findings from this study are in contrast to those from the study by Goldzieher and colleagues (1971a, 1971b), which found mood worsening most pronounced when the OC administered was high in estrogen and progestin. The Cullberg (1972) study does not support a dose relationship between the amount of progestin and the degree of mood changes: for some measures, mood changes were greatest in the lower-dose progestin group and lowest in the intermediate-dose progestin group, whereas for other measures, the reverse was true. Because there was no progestin-only group for comparison, it could not be determined whether estrogen was contributing to the mood changes.

A third placebo-controlled OC study (Graham et al. 1995) was conducted in two countries (Edinburgh, Scotland and Manila, Philippines), with each center including 25 women in each of three treatment conditions: placebo, combined ethinyl estradiol (0.03 mg/day) and levonorgestrel (0.15 mg/day), or progestin-only therapy (levonorgestrel 0.03 mg/day). Women received treatment for 4 months, and mood was monitored with the Beck Depression Inventory (Beck et al. 1961). In both centers, women in the progestin-only group showed a mild reduction in mood symptoms, whereas at the Manila site, the degree of depression increased in women given either placebo or combined OCs. There was a significant difference between treatment groups for the combined centers, but the greatest difference seen was for "wellness": the progestin group had by far the greatest improvement in this measure. Again, this study does not support significant mood worsening associated with OCs, since the combined-OC group was similar to the placebo group and the progestin-only group fared better than the other groups.

The effects of OCs on mood were also assessed in women with PMS (Graham and Sherwin 1993). An OC with sequential increase of progestin was used in this clinical trial. Whereas similar mood effects were reported by women receiving the OC and women receiving placebo during the the premenstrual phase of the cycle, women on the OC had more mood symptoms than women on placebo during the early follicular phase, when progestin doses were lowest.

These results show limited support for OC-induced mood deterioration. With some outcome measures used in the Cullberg (1972) and the Graham and Sherwin (1993) studies, mood worsening was more likely to occur in women receiving the lowest dose of progestin in combination with estrogen. One possible explanation for this puzzling finding is that a relatively higher dose of progestin is needed to provide some protection against the mood-worsening effects of estrogen. On the other hand, Gold-zieher and colleagues (1971a, 1971b) found that the women in their trial fared least well when they took higher-dose hormonal preparations. However, it may be that when estrogen is given at higher doses, such as in the Goldzieher et al. (1971a, 1971b) study, the progestin may not be able to counteract the estrogen's deleterious effects on mood. Some support is found for this latter proposition in the older study by de Lignieres and Vincens (1982), reviewed above. These researchers found that estrogen was associated with a dose-related increase in anxiety symptoms that could be improved with progesterone administration.

Treatment Recommendations

Women who undergo surgical menopause are the population that most consistently benefits from estrogen therapy. The data showing benefit for estrogen are quite consistent, and the type of estrogen preparation employed does not appear to matter. A change in estrogen preparation should be considered if a woman fails to respond to conjugated estrogens or to other preparations that predominantly deliver estrone, and if there are no contraindications to parenteral or transdermal estrogen.

Data suggest that women who are naturally menopausal are also likely to derive mood-elevating benefits from estrogen administration, particularly if the estrogen is 17 β-estradiol. Data also suggest that estrogen therapy alleviates mood symptoms in perimenopausal women and that it may actually be more effective in this group than in postmenopausal women. One study of perimenopausal women with particularly severe MDD symptoms (Schmidt et al. [submitted for publication]) found that estrogen was effective in this group. In contrast, estrogen was not superior to placebo for treating MDD in postmenopausal women in another study (Saletu et al. 1995). Studies of estrogen treatment for MDD that is not reproductive related suggest only modest clinical benefit for estrogen as monotherapy. Certainly, HRT should be considered for other reasons (maintenance of bone, protection against coronary artery and cerebrovascular disease), but it should not be relied upon as a routine treatment for MDD as well.

Clinicians should not be wary of using OCs in women because of mood-lowering effects. It is likely that if a mood disorder occurs, it would have occurred in any case and may be due to psychosocial factors rather than hormonal factors. One study has suggested that women with severe PMS are sensitive to changing levels of endogenous hormones and may be at risk for mood deterioration if hormonal therapies are administered (Graham and Sherwin 1993). However, another study found that an earlier diagnosis of PMS did not influence the induction of mood symptoms in postmenopausal women (Kirkham et al. 1991). Moreover, non-placebo-controlled studies have shown that women with PMS may benefit from OCs (Backstrom et al. 1992; Walker and Bancroft 1990). Many women reporting severe PMS actually have another psychiatric condition or mood symptoms unrelated to the luteal phase of the menstrual cycle (Rubinow and Roy-Byrne 1984). Thus, retrospective reports of PMS should not deter clinicians from the routine use of OCs.

Summary

There is support for the contention that estrogen alleviates milder mood disturbances in peri- and postmenopausal women, but there is little support for the view that progestins cause mood worsening. The estrogen preparations most strongly associated with positive mood changes include percutaneous and transdermal preparations delivering 17 β-estradiol. It may be that some of the differences in response among the various studies are due to the type of estrogen used.

In terms of the effects of OCs on mood, the widely held belief that OCs induce negative mood changes is not uniformly supported and should not be quoted as fact. Rather, results from placebo-controlled trials favor the findings of a large British epidemiological study of more than 16,000 women (Vessey et al. 1985) that showed no difference in mood symptoms among women using OCs, a diaphragm, or an intrauterine device.

References

Aylward M, Holly F, Parker RJ: An evaluation of clinical response to piperazine-oestrone sulphate ("Harmogen") in menopausal patients. Curr Med Res Opin 2:417–423, 1974

Backstrom T: Symptoms related to the menopause and sex steroid treatments. Ciba Found Symp 191:171–186, 1995

Backstrom T, Hansson-Malmstrom Y, Lindhe B-A, et al: Oral contraceptives in premenstrual syndrome: a randomized comparison of triphasic and monophasic preparations. Contraception 46:253–268, 1992

Ballinger CB: Psychiatric morbidity and the menopause: screening of general population sample. BMJ 3:344–346, 1975

Ballinger CB: Psychiatric aspects of the menopause. Br J Psychiatry 156:773–787, 1990

Barrett-Connor E, Kritz-Silverstein D: Estrogen replacement therapy and cognitive function in older women. JAMA 269:2637–2641, 1993

Beck A, Ward C, Mendelson M, et al: An inventory for measuring depression. Arch Gen Psychiatry 42:667–675, 1961

Biegon A, Reches A, Snyder L, et al: Serotonergic and noradrenergic receptors in the rat brain: modulation by chronic exposure to ovarian hormones. Life Sci 32:2015–2021, 1983

Bitran D, Purdy RH, Kellogg CK: Anxiolytic effect of progesterone is associated with increases in cortical allopregnanolone and $GABA_A$ receptor function. Pharmacol Biochem Behav 45:423–428, 1993

Brincat M, Studd JWW, O'Dowd T, et al: Subcutaneous hormone implants for the control of climacteric symptoms. Lancet 7:16–18, 1984

Bullock JL, Massey FM, Gambrell RD: Use of medroxyprogesterone acetate to prevent menopausal symptoms. Obstet Gynecol 46:165–168, 1975

Bungay GT, Vessey MP, McPherson CK: Study of symptoms in middle life with special reference to the menopause. BMJ 281:181–183, 1980

Campbell S: Double blind psychometric studies on the effects of natural estrogens on post-menopausal women, in The Management of Menopause and Postmenopausal Years. Edited by Campbell S. Baltimore, MD, University Park Press, MTP, 1976, pp 149–158

Campbell S, Whitehead M: Oestrogen therapy and the menopausal syndrome. Clin Obstet Gynaecol 4:31–47, 1977

Coope J: The menopause: is oestrogen therapy effective in the treatment of menopausal depression? Journal of the Royal College of General Practitioners 31:134–140, 1981

Coope J, Thomson JM, Poller L: Effects of "natural oestrogen" replacement therapy on menopausal symptoms and blood clotting. BMJ 4:139–143, 1975

Coppen A, Bishop M, Beard RJ: Effects of piperazine oestrone sulphate on plasma tryptophan, oestrogens, gonadotrophins and psychological functioning in women following hysterectomy. Curr Med Res Opin 4:29–36, 1977

Cullberg J: Mood changes and menstrual symptoms with different gestagen/estrogen combinations: a double blind comparison with a placebo. Acta Psychiatr Scand Suppl 236:1–86, 1972

Dalton K: Prospective study into puerperal depression. Br J Psychiatry 118:689–692, 1971

de Lignieres B, Vincens M: Differential effects of exogenous oestradiol and progesterone on mood in post-menopausal women: individual dose/effect relationship. Maturitas 4:67–72, 1982

Dennerstein L: Mood and menopause, in The Menopause and Hormonal Replacement Therapy: Facts and Controversies. Edited by Sitruk-Ware R, Utian WH. New York, Marcel Dekker, 1991, pp 101–118

Dennerstein L, Burrows GD: Affect and the menstrual cycle. J Affect Disord 1:77–92, 1979

Derman RJ, Dawood MY, Stone S: Quality of life during sequential hormone replacement therapy: a placebo-controlled study. International Journal of Fertility 40:73–78, 1995

Dhar V, Murphy BEP: Double-blind randomized crossover trial of luteal phase estrogens (Premarin) in the premenstrual syndrome (PMS). Psychoneuroendocrinology 15:489–493, 1991

Dickerson J, Bressler R, Christian CD, et al: Efficacy of estradiol vaginal cream in postmenopausal women. Clin Pharmacol Ther 26:502–507, 1979

Ditkoff EC, Crary WG, Cristo M, et al: Estrogen improves psychological function in asymptomatic postmenopausal women. Obstet Gynecol 78:991–995, 1991

Fedor-Freybergh P: The influence of oestrogen on well-being and mental performance in climacteric postmenopausal women. Acta Obstet Gynecol Scand 64:1–91, 1977

Fink G, Sumner BE, Rosie R, et al: Estrogen control of central neurotransmission: effect on mood, mental state, and memory. Cell Mol Neurobiol 16:325–344, 1996

Fischette CT, Biegon A, McEwen BS: Sex differences in serotonin 1 receptor binding in rat brain. Science 222:333–335, 1983

Freeman EW, Purdy RH, Coutifaris C, et al: Anxiolytic metabolites of progesterone: correlation with mood and performance measures following oral progesterone administration to healthy female volunteers. Neuroendocrinology 58:478–484, 1993

Furuhjelm M, Karlgren E, Carlstrom K: The effect of estrogen therapy on somatic and psychical symptoms in postmenopausal women. Acta Obstet Gynecol Scand 63:655–666, 1984

George GCW, Utian WH, Beumont PJV, et al: Effect of exogenous oestrogens on minor psychiatric symptoms in postmenopausal women. S Afr Med J 47:2387–2388, 1973

Gerdes LC, Sonnendecker EWW, Polakow ES: Psychological changes effected by estrogen–progestogen and clonidine treatment in climacteric women. Am J Obstet Gynecol 142:98–104, 1982

Gereau RW IV, Kedzie KA, Renner KJ: Effect of progesterone on serotonin turnover in rats primed with estrogen implants into the ventromedial hypothalamus. Brain Res Bull 32:293–300, 1993

Goldzieher JW, Moses LE, Averkin E, et al: A placebo-controlled double-blind crossover investigation of the side effects attributed to oral contraceptives. Fertil Steril 22:609–623, 1971a

Goldzieher JW, Moses LE, Averkin E, et al: Nervousness and depression attributed to oral contraceptives: a double-blind, placebo-controlled study. Am J Obstet Gynecol 111:1013–1020, 1971b

Graham CA, Sherwin BB: The relationship between mood and sexuality in women using an oral contraceptive as a treatment for premenstrual symptoms. Psychoneuroendocrinology 8:273–281, 1993

Graham CA, Ramos R, Bancroft J, et al: The effects of steroidal contraceptives on the well-being and sexuality of women: a double-blind, placebo-controlled, two-centre study of combined and progestogen-only methods. Contraception 52:363–369, 1995

Gregoire AJ, Kumar R, Everitt B, et al: Transdermal oestrogen for treatment of severe postnatal depression. Lancet 347:930–933, 1996

Halbreich U: Role of estrogen in postmenopausal depression. Neurology 48 (suppl 7):S16–S20, 1997

Halbreich U, Lumley LA: The multiple interactional biological processes that might lead to depression and gender differences in its appearance. J Affect Disord 29:159–173, 1993

Halbreich U, Rojansky N, Palter S, et al: Estrogen augments serotonergic activity in postmenopausal women. Biol Psychiatry 37:434–441, 1995

Hallstrom T, Samuelsson S: Mental health in the climacteric: the longitudinal study of women in Gothenburg. Acta Obstet Gynecol Scand Suppl 130:13–18, 1985

Hamilton M: A rating scale for depression. J Neurol Neurosurg Psychiatry 23:56–62, 1960

Hammarback S, Backstrom T, Holst J, et al: Cyclical mood changes as in the premenstrual tension syndrome during sequential estrogen–progestogen postmenopausal replacement therapy. Acta Obstet Gynecol Scand 64:393–397, 1985

Holst J, Backstrom T, Hammarback S, et al: Progestogen addition during oestrogen replacement therapy: effects on vasomotor symptoms and mood. Maturitas 11:13–20, 1989

Hunter M, Battersby R, Whitehead M: Relationships between psychological symptoms, somatic complaints and menopausal status. Maturitas 8:217–228, 1986

Jones EE, Naftolin F: Estrogen effects on the tuberoinfundibular dopaminergic system in the female rat brain. Brain Res 510:84–91, 1990

Kampen DL, Sherwin BB: Estrogen use and verbal memory in healthy postmenopausal women. Obstet Gynecol 83:979–983, 1994

Kaufert PA, Gilbert P, Tate R: The Manitoba Project: a re-examination of the link between menopause and depression. Maturitas 14:143–155, 1992

Kirkham C, Hahn PM, Van Vugt DA, et al: A randomized, double-blind, placebo-controlled, cross-over trial to assess the side effects of medroxyprogesterone acetate in hormone replacement therapy. Obstet Gynecol 78:93–97, 1991

Klaiber EL, Broverman DM, Vogel W, et al: Estrogen therapy for severe persistent depressions in women. Arch Gen Psychiatry 36:550–554, 1979

Klaiber EL, Broverman DM, Vogel W, et al: Individual differences in changes in mood and platelet monoamine oxidase (MAO) activity during hormonal replacement therapy in menopausal women. Psychoneuroendocrinology 21:575–592, 1996

Lobo RA (ed): Preface, in Treatment of the Postmenopausal Woman: Basic and Clinical Aspects. New York, Lippincott-Raven, 1994, pp 15–20

Lyman GW, Johnson RN: Assay for conjugated estrogens in tablets using fused-silica capillary gas chromatography. J Chromatogr A 234:234–239, 1982

Magos AL, Brewster E, Singh R, et al: The effects of norethisterone in postmenopausal women on oestrogen replacement therapy: a model for the premenstrual syndrome. Br J Obstet Gynaecol 93:1290–1296, 1986

Mahesh VB, Brann DW, Hendry LB: Diverse modes of action of progesterone and its metabolites. J Steroid Biochem Mol Biol 56:209–219, 1996

Majewska MD, Harrison NZ, Schwartz RD, et al: Steroid hormone metabolites are barbiturate-like modulators of the GABA receptor. Science 252:1001–1007, 1986

Maoz B, Durst N: The effects of oestrogen therapy on the sex life of post-menopausal women. Maturitas 2:327–336, 1980

Matthews KA: Myths and realities of the menopause. Psychosom Med 54:1–9, 1992

McKinlay JB, McKinlay SM, Brambilla D: The relative contributions of endocrine changes and social circumstances to depression in mid-aged women. J Health Soc Behav 28:345–363, 1987

McReynolds P: The Hospital Adjustment Scale: research and clinical applications. Psychol Rep 23:823–835, 1968

Michael CM, Kantor HI, Shore H: Further psychometric evaluation of older women—the effect of estrogen administration. Journal of Gerontology 25:337–341, 1970

Montgomery JC, Brincat M, Tapp A, et al: Effect of oestrogen and testosterone implants on psychological disorders in the climacteric. Lancet 7:297–299, 1987

Moos RH: The development of a menstrual distress questionnaire. Psychosom Med 30:853–867, 1968

Morrison JC, Martin DC, Blair RA, et al: The use of medroxyprogesterone acetate for relief of climacteric symptoms. Am J Obstet Gynecol 138:99–104, 1980

O'Keane V, O'Hanlon M, Webb M, et al T: D-fenfluramine/prolactin response throughout the menstrual cycle: evidence for an oestrogen-induced alteration. Clin Endocrinol (Oxf) 34:289–292, 1991

Palinkas LA, Barrett-Connor E: Estrogen use and depressive symptoms in postmenopausal women. Obstet Gynecol 80:30–36, 1992

Paterson MEL: A randomized, double-blind, cross-over study into the effect of sequential mestranol and norethisterone on climacteric symptoms and biochemical parameters. Maturitas 4:83–94, 1982

Pecins-Thompson M, Brown NA, Kohama SG, et al: Ovarian steroid regulation of tryptophan hydroxylase mRNA expression in rhesus macaques. J Neurosci 16:7021–7029, 1996

Phillips SM, Sherwin BB: Effects of estrogen on memory function in surgically menopausal women. Psychoneuroendocrinology 17:485–495, 1992

Prange AJ, Lipton MA, Nemeroff CB, et al: The role of hormones in depression. Life Sci 20:1305–1318, 1977

Prior JC, Alojado N, McKay DW, et al: No adverse effects of medroxyprogesterone treatment without estrogen in postmenopausal women: double-blind, placebo-controlled, crossover trial. Obstet Gynecol 83:24–28, 1994

Rojansky N, Halbreich U, Zander K, et al: Imipramine receptor binding and serotonin uptake in platelets of women with premenstrual changes. Gynecol Obstet Invest 31:146–152, 1991

Rubinow DR, Roy-Byrne P: Premenstrual syndromes: overview from a methodologic perspective. Am J Psychiatry 141:163–172, 1984

Saletu B, Brandstatter N, Metka M, et al: Double-blind, placebo-controlled, hormonal, syndromal and EEG mapping studies with transdermal oestradiol therapy in menopausal depression. Psychopharmacology 122:321–329, 1995

Schmidt PJ, Nieman LK, Danaceau MA, Tobin MB, Roca CA, Murphy JH, Rubinow DR: Estrogen replacement in perimenopause-related depression. Am J Obstet Gynecol (submitted for publication)

Schneider LS, Small GW, Hamilton SH, et al: Estrogen replacement and response to fluoxetine in a multicenter geriatric depression trial (The Fluoxetine Collaborative Study Group). Am J Geriatr Psychiatry 5:97–106, 1997

Schneider LS, Small GW, Clary C: Estrogen replacement therapy status and antidepressant response to sertraline. Paper presented at the 151st Annual Meeting of the American Psychiatric Association, Toronto, Ontario, Canada, May 1998

Shapira B, Oppenheim G, Zohar J, et al: Lack of efficacy of estrogen supplementation to imipramine in resistant female depressives. Biol Psychiatry 20:576–579, 1985

Sherwin BB: The impact of different doses of estrogen and progestin on mood and sexual behavior in postmenopausal women. J Clin Endocrinol Metab 72:336–343, 1991

Sherwin BB: Estrogenic effects on memory in women. Ann N Y Acad Sci 743:213–230, 1994

Sherwin BB, Gelfand MM: Sex steroids and affect in the surgical menopause: a double-blind, cross-over study. Psychoneuroendocrinology 10:325–335, 1985

Sherwin BB, Gelfand MM, Brender W: Androgen enhances sexual motivation in females: a prospective, crossover study of sex steroid administration in the surgical menopause. Psychosom Med 47:339–351, 1985

Shimizu H, Bray GA: Effects of castration, estrogen replacement and estrus cycle on monoamine metabolism in the nucleus accumbens, measured by microdialysis. Brain Res 721:200–206, 1993

Slap GB: Oral contraceptives and depression: impact, prevalence and cause. Journal of Adolescent Health Care 2:53–64, 1981

Smith SS: Female sex steroid hormones from receptors to networks to performance: actions on the sensorimotor system. Prog Neurobiol 44:55–86, 1994

Stanczyk FZ, Shoupe D, Nunez V, et al: A randomized comparison of hormonal estradiol delivery in postmenopausal women. Am J Obstet Gynecol 159:1540–1546, 1988

Steiner M, Lepage P, Dunn EJ: Serotonin and gender-specific psychiatric disorders. International Journal of Psychiatry in Clinical Practice 1:3–13, 1997

Steiner M, Yonkers KA, Eriksson E: Depression in Women. London, Martin Dunitz Ltd, 1998

Strickler RC, Borth R, Cecutti A, et al: The role of oestrogen replacement in the climacteric syndrome. Psychol Med 7:631–639, 1977

Studd JWW, Smith RNJ: Estrogens and depression in women. Menopause [The Journal of the North American Menopause Society] 1: 33–37, 1994

Studd J, Chakravarti S, Oram D: The climacteric. Clin Obstet Gynaecol 4:3–29, 1977

Stuenkel CA: Menopause and estrogen replacement therapy. Psychiatr Clin North Am 2:133–152, 1989

Sumner BEH, Fink G: Estrogen increases the density of 5-hydroxytryptamine-2A receptors in cerebral cortex and nucleus accumbens in the female rat. J Steroid Biochem Mol Biol 54:15–20, 1995

Thomson J, Oswald I: Effect of oestrogen on the sleep, mood, and anxiety of menopausal women. BMJ 2:1317–1319, 1977

Vessey MP, McPherson K, Lawless M, et al: Oral contraception and serious psychiatric illness: absence of an association. Br J Psychiatry 146:45–49, 1985

Walker A, Bancroft J: Relationship between premenstrual symptoms and oral contraceptive use: a controlled study. Psychosom Med 52: 86–96, 1990

Watson NR, Judd JWW, Savvas M, et al: Treatment of severe premenstrual syndrome with oestradiol patches and cyclical oral norethisterone. Lancet 335:730–732, 1989

Whitehead MI, Hillard TC, Crook D: The role and use of progestogens. Obstet Gynecol 75:59S–76S, 1990

Wiklund I, Karlberg J, Mattsson LA: Quality of life of postmenopausal women on a regimen of transdermal estradiol therapy: a double-blind placebo-controlled study. Am J Obstet Gynecol 168:824–830, 1993

Yonkers KA, Bradshaw K: Estrogens, progestins and mood, in Mood Disorders in Women. Edited by Steiner M, Yonkers KA, Eriksson E. London, Martin Dunitz Ltd (in press)

Zuckerman M, Lubin B: Multiple Adjective Affect Checklist: Manual. San Diego, CA, EdITS, 1965

Zweifel JE, O'Brien WH: A meta-analysis of the effect of hormone replacement therapy upon depressed mood. Psychoneuroendocrinology 22:189–212, 1997

Chapter 5

Modulation of Monoamine Neurotransmitters by Estrogen: Clinical Implications

Charles DeBattista, M.D., D.M.H.,
David Lawrence Smith, M.D., and
Alan F. Schatzberg, M.D.

In recent years, the complex interaction of estrogen and mono-amine neurotransmitters has been increasingly appreciated. Estrogen appears to have specific and significant effects on serotonin (5-hydroxytryptamine [5-HT]), dopamine (DA), norepinephrine (NE), and monoamine oxidase (MAO). The effects of estrogen on monoamines may explain some of the gender differences seen in the clinical presentation and treatment response of disorders such as major depression and schizophrenia. Estrogen's monoamine effects also suggest a potential role in the treatment of some mood and psychotic disorders.

Estrogen Modulation of Serotonin

Serotonin has been implicated to have a central role in many psychiatric disorders, especially major depression. Many lines of evidence suggest that estrogen modulates serotonergic function, including synthesis, receptor binding, and synaptic uptake (Table 5–1).

The effects of estrogen on 5-HT synthesis appear to be dose and time specific. In the rat dorsal raphe, estrogen appears to increase the level and synthesis of 5-HT. However, in the rat hypothala-

Table 5–1. Summary of neurochemical studies of estrogen modulation of serotonin (5-HT)

Neurotransmitter effect	Estrogen condition	Finding	Study
5-HT synthesis	Acute estradiol	Increased synthesis	Cone et al. 1981
5-HT receptors	Acute estradiol, chronic estradiol	Increased 5-HT$_2$, decreased 5-HT$_1$	Biegon and McEwen 1982; Clarke and Goldfarb 1989; Fink et al. 1996
Imipramine binding	Acute estradiol, menstrual variation	Increased imipramine binding	Rojansky et al. 1991; Stockert and DeRobertis 1985
5-HT reuptake	Acute estradiol, menstrual variation	Increased reuptake, no change	Endersby and Wilson 1974; Tam et al. 1985; Wirz-Justice et al. 1974

Note. 5-HT = 5-hydroxytryptamine (serotonin).

mus, estradiol injection causes an increase in 5-hydroxyindole-acetic acid (5-HIAA), but not 5-HT, levels. Cone and colleagues (1981) examined brain regions in ovariectomized rats and intact controls following administration of estradiol and progesterone. After the administration of ovarian steroids, 5-HT levels increased in the median and mesencephalic raphe nuclei of the ovariectomized animals but not in other parts of the rat brain. Because most 5-HT synthesis takes place in the raphe, this finding was not unexpected. However, no significant increases in 5-HT levels were noted in the control animals.

Likewise, estrogen appears to exert significant modulatory effects on 5-HT receptors. Animal studies have demonstrated that estrogen may be necessary in the downregulation of 5-HT receptors that is seen after antidepressant administration. Kendell and colleagues (1987) demonstrated that ovariectomized rats failed to downregulate 5-HT receptors in response to administration of a tricyclic antidepressant (TCA). However, downregulation was established when estradiol was added to the TCA. Similarly, Biegon and McEwen (1982) found a biphasic effect of estrogen on the density of 5-HT receptors throughout the brain. The administration of estrogen to female rats resulted in a reduction in 5-HT receptors throughout the brain, followed by a selective increase 48–72 hours later in regions of the brain including the preoptic area, hypothalamus, and amygdala. Biegon and McEwen concluded that estrogen had both an immediate effect on neuron membranes to modify 5-HT receptor availability and a slower effect that was more anatomically specific.

Studies suggest that estrogen may act on specific receptors, including 5-HT$_{2A}$ and 5-HT$_1$, which are thought to play a critical role in depression and anxiety, among other disorders. Furthermore, acute administration of estrogen may cause different effects on 5-HT receptor density than chronic administration. For example, Fink et al. (1996) has demonstrated that *chronic* estrogen administration stimulated an increase in density of 5-HT$_2$ receptors in the anterior frontal cortex, cingulate cortex, nucleus accumbens, and primary olfactory cortex. Because these anatomic regions are thought to be important in the mediation of mood, behavior, and cognition, some of estrogen's potential therapeutic benefits may be directly related to its 5-HT$_2$ effects.

Estrogen also decreases 5-HT$_1$ receptors in ovariectomized rats, while progesterone may block those effects when given concurrently (Biegon and McEwen 1982). In the rat hippocampus, estrogen increases the sensitivity of 5-HT$_{1A}$ receptors (Clarke and Goldfarb 1989).

Imipramine binding and 5-HT platelet binding are thought to reflect central serotonin activity, and a number of animal studies have suggested that estrogen may have profound effects on these measures of 5-HT activity in the brain. In a study of ovariectomized rats, Stockert and DeRobertis (1985) reported that [^{3}H]imipramine receptor binding increased by 200% in ovariectomized rats. Human studies have also suggested that changes in platelet binding are strongly influenced by levels of ovarian hormones during different parts of the menstrual cycle. In women with a history of premenstrual dysphoria, imipramine binding was lower in the early luteal phase, before they developed symptoms, than it was in control women without premenstrual mood changes (Rojansky et al. 1991).

The synaptic reuptake of 5-HT is influenced to some extent by estrogen (Endersby and Wilson 1974; Wirz-Justice et al. 1974); in rat studies, changes in estradiol levels during the estrous cycle were directly correlated with hypothalamic 5-HT uptake. Likewise, injection of estradiol results in time-, region-, and dose-specific changes in 5-HT reuptake. Human studies have been less consistent than animal models in showing a direct correlation between 5-HT reuptake and estrogen. For example, in a study by Tam and colleagues (1985), no correlation was found between phase of the menstrual cycle, mood, and platelet 5-HT reuptake.

If estrogen enhances central serotonin activity, it might also be expected that estrogen would augment serotonergic drugs. This appears to be the case. Halbreich et al. (1995) examined the 5-HT$_2$ agonist meta-chlorphenylpiperazine (m-CPP) in a study of 18 postmenopausal women. They found that the typical prolactin and cortisol response to m-CPP was blunted. However, when the women were treated with an estrogen patch (0.1 mg), the prolactin and cortisol response normalized, which suggests that estrogen may augment the effects of 5-HT agonists. Another possibility, however, is that estrogen was directly stimulating prolactin and was not acting indirectly through serotonergic mechanisms.

Thus, there may be a direct correlation between deficiencies in estrogen—whether resulting from hysterectomy, from changes in the menstrual cycle, or from menopause—and deficiencies in 5-HT level or function. The clinical relevance of this correlation, and the role of estrogen's serotonergic effects in the pathophysiology of mood and anxiety disorders, remains to be determined; the current state of our knowledge is discussed in Chapter 2 in this volume.

Estrogen Modulation of Dopamine

Estrogen appears to modulate the neurotransmission of DA as significantly as it does that of 5-HT. Evidence for estrogen's influence on DA comes both directly from neurochemical and behavioral studies and indirectly from studies of the relationship between psychotic disorders and estrogen levels in humans.

Many studies have demonstrated at a biochemical level that estrogen influences DA receptor affinity and number, as well as DA neurotransmitter concentration and release, although the direction of change varies, depending on several factors, including the estrogen dosage used, the length of time of administration, and the particular brain region examined (Van Hartesveldt and Joyce 1986).

Häfner et al. (1993) studied the effect of chronic estradiol administration on the striatum of ovariectomized rats and found a 2.8-fold reduction in dopamine-2 (D_2) receptor affinity as measured by radiolabeled sulpiride. A decrease in D_2 receptor affinity has also been found in ovariectomized rats after acute administration of estradiol (Gordon and Perry 1983). However, the actual number of DA receptors has been shown to increase in response to estrogen treatment, once again in ovariectomized rats (Hruska and Silbergeld 1980).

Estrogen also influences other aspects of DA transmission, including turnover and release, although, again, the direction of change is affected by dosage and region examined. Di Paolo et al. (1985) found that acute estrogen administration rapidly increased DA turnover. After injecting ovariectomized rats with 17 β-estradiol, these investigators noted an increase in two DA metabolites, dehydroxyphenylacetic acid and homovanillic acid, an effect that occurred 30 minutes after injection and that coincided with peak estradiol concentrations. Increases in striatal DA release in response to acute estrogen administration have been directly measured by other authors (Becker 1990; Xiao and Becker 1998). Chronic estrogen treatment, however, seems to have an effect opposite to that of acute administration: Dupont et al. (1981) showed that DA concentrations were significantly reduced in several brain nuclei in ovariectomized rats under conditions of chronic estrogen treatment, although DA turnover was unaffected. Finally, Morissette and Di Paolo (1993) found that chronic exposure to either estradiol or progesterone increased DA uptake site density, a component of DA turnover, in the nigrostriatal dopamine system but not in the nucleus accumbens or the substantia nigra pars reticulata. The neurochemical evidence for estrogen's effect on DA neurotransmission is summarized in Table 5–2.

Table 5–2. Summary of neurochemical studies of estrogen modulation of dopamine (DA)

Neurotransmitter effect	Estrogen condition	Finding	Study
DA D_2 receptor affinity	Acute estradiol	Decreased receptor affinity	Gordon and Perry 1983
	Chronic estradiol	Decreased receptor affinity	Häfner et al. 1991
DA D_2 receptor number	Chronic estradiol	Decreased number of receptors	Hruska and Silbergeld 1980
DA turnover	Acute estradiol	Increased turnover	Di Paolo et al. 1985
	Chronic estradiol	No change noted	Dupont et al. 1981
DA concentration and release	Acute estradiol	Increased release as measured by increase in DA metabolites	Di Paolo et al. 1985
		Increased release directly measured	Becker 1990; Xiao and Becker 1998
	Chronic estradiol	Decreased concentration in several brain nuclei	Dupont et al. 1981
		Increased DA uptake site density in nigrostriatal system	Morissette and Di Paolo 1993

In addition to the neurochemical data, there exists a significant body of animal studies demonstrating that estrogen can influence behaviors understood to be mediated by DA centers in the brain. In most of these studies, estrogen acts much like a typical neuroleptic, both by decreasing the manifestation of behaviors related to DA agonism and by enhancing manifestations of DA blockade. In rats, estrogen reduces DA-related circling behavior (Bedard et al. 1978); it also decreases locomotion frequency, reduces stereotypies (i.e., downward sniffing, licking/chewing, sitting, and grooming behaviors) provoked by the DA agonists amphetamine and apomorphine, and worsens catalepsy induced by neuroleptics (Palermo-Neto and Dorce 1990).

Estrogen's effects, however, are not limited to blocking the behavioral manifestations of DA activity; it appears also to *enhance* these manifestations, again depending on the dosage and chronicity of its administration. Bedard et al. (1985), using a monkey model for tardive dyskinesia in which a midbrain lesion produced lingual dyskinesia, found that when given in small doses, estradiol acutely increased dyskinesia, whereas large doses led to decreased dyskinesia. Additional evidence for the ability of estrogen to enhance DA neurotransmission comes from Nausieda et al. (1979), who showed that chronic estradiol treatment restores amphetamine- and apomorphine-induced stereotypies in ovariectomized guinea pigs, and from Hruska and Silbergeld (1980), who found that the duration of amphetamine-induced rotation in rats previously treated with the neurotoxin 6-hydroxydopamine increased from 81 to 106 seconds 5–8 days after a single estradiol injection. One explanation for estrogen's apparent biphasic effects on DA transmission is that it acutely reduces DA activity, thereby provoking a compensatory upregulation in postsynaptic DA receptors, much as is theorized to be the case with the development of tardive dyskinesia in humans after chronic neuroleptic treatment. Such an explanation is supported by data from Harrer and Schmidt (1986), who treated male ferrets with estrogen for 3 days. Compared with controls, the estrogen-treated ferrets demonstrated increased apomorphine-induced stereotypies 2–3 days after estrogen discontinuation.

Despite the somewhat contradictory evidence that estrogen

has the ability both to reduce and to enhance DA neurotrans-mission, all of the studies of estrogen's effects on DA described here agree that estrogen significantly modulates the DA system. Although it is not known how estrogen interacts at the molecular level with the DA system to produce its many demonstrated biochemical and behavioral effects, several possible mechanisms may be operative.

One mechanism by which estrogen influences DA neurons is by binding to an intracellular steroid receptor, thereby affecting genomic functions. Guivarc'h et al. (1995) showed that estradiol binds to intracellular receptors in the olfactory tubercule and hy-pothalamus but not in the striatum, which has been found not to express intracellular estrogen receptors. In agreement with this localization, Guivarc'h and colleagues also found that estrogen treatment modulated the splicing of two isoforms on the D_2 re-ceptor in the olfactory tubercule and hypothalamus but not in the striatum. Another demonstrated genomic effect of estrogen is a decrease in the rate of tyrosine hydroxylase gene transcription in tuberoinfundibular neurons (Blum et al. 1987).

A second mechanism by which estrogen may modulate the ac-tivity of DA neurons is by binding to an extracellular membrane-bound receptor, with consequent effects on G protein and sec-ond-messenger systems. This mechanism may better explain the striatally based behavioral changes noted in animals, because estrogen's behavioral effects occur too quickly to be attributed to genomic modulation, and striatal DA neurons in this region do not concentrate estrogen intracellularly (Simerly et al. 1990). Evidence for a membrane-bound estrogen receptor has recently been found in striatal cells: Mermelstein et al. (1996) used whole-cell-clamp recording techniques to show that the β isomer of 17 estradiol was much more effective than the α isomer in reduc-ing calcium current in striatal neurons, an effect that occurred within milliseconds. To further demonstrate that the β isomer was causing these changes by acting extracellularly, Mermelstein and colleagues conjugated the β isomer with bovine serum albu-min (BSA), which prevents the isomer's entry into the neuron, and found an equal reduction in calcium current; when G protein inactivation was inhibited, this effect was prolonged. Similarly,

Xiao and Becker (1998) tested different agents, all known to be agonists of the intracellular steroid receptor, for their effectiveness in enhancing amphetamine-stimulated DA release in ovariectomized rats. They hypothesized that a membrane-bound estrogen receptor would have a different stereospecificity than the intracellular receptor and, thus, that they would find differential effects on DA release. Indeed, 4- and 2-hydroxyestradiol enhanced DA release, but estrone, estriol, and diethylstilbestrol did not. Additionally, the estradiol–BSA conjugate (which again is prevented from entering the neuron) also enhanced DA release. These data further confirm the presence of a specific membrane-binding site for estrogen in the striatum.

A third potential mechanism for estrogen's modulation of DA neurotransmission may be indirect, via estrogen's influence on the 5-HT system. As reviewed by Kapur and Remington (1996), several systems of DA neurons exhibit 5-HT_2 heteroreceptors that inhibit the DA neurons' function so that an increase in serotonergic activity at 5-HT_2 receptors leads to a decrease in DA neurotransmission. In fact, 5-HT_2 blockade and the consequent increase in nigrostriatal DA transmission is one mechanism thought to confer upon atypical antipsychotics a lower risk of extrapyramidal side effects than is seen with typical antipsychotics, which lack 5-HT_2 antagonism.

Estrogen Modulation of Norepinephrine

The modulation of NE by estrogen is somewhat less well studied than estrogen's effects on 5-HT and DA. However, over the past 25 years, data have accumulated that suggest an important role for estrogen and other ovarian steroids in the modulation of NE (Table 5–3). Thus, there has been an interest in the interrelation of NE and estrogen in women's mood disorders. As is the case with other monoamines, estrogen may play a role in every phase of NE activity, including synthesis, release, adrenergic receptor activity, and enzymatic degradation.

The rate-limiting enzyme in the synthesis of catecholamines, NE included, is tyrosine hydroxylase, whereas the catecholamines are metabolized by MAO. As reported earlier in this

Table 5–3. Summary of neurochemical studies of estrogen modulation of norepinephrine (NE)

Neurotransmitter effect	Estrogen condition	Finding	Study
NE synthesis	Acute estradiol	Decrease or increase	Etgen and Karkanias 1994; Paul et al. 1979
α_2 activity	Menstrual, menopause, postpartum	Estrogen antagonizes	Jones et al. 1983; Kuevi et al. 1983; Metz et al. 1983
MHPG	Estradiol implant, menopause	Increased MHPG, decreased MHPG	Best et al. 1992; Halbreich and Lumley 1993

Note. MHPG = 3-methoxy-4-hydroxyphenylethyleneglycol.

chapter, estrogen appears to differentially inhibit tyrosine hydroxylase and MAO in different regions of the brain. Therefore, estrogen affects both the synthesis and the metabolism of NE (Janowsky et al. 1971).

Several lines of evidence suggest that estrogen may tonically enhance NE release in both animals and humans. Paul and colleagues (1979) used short-term organ cultures of rat hypothalamus to study the effects of various estrogenic compounds on catecholamine release. They found a direct correlation between the dosage of potent estrogenic compounds, such as 17 β-estradiol and diethylstilbestrol, and catecholamine release from the hypothalamus. Weak estrogenic compounds, such as estrone and estriol, failed to stimulate efflux of NE from the hypothalamus. These findings are consistent with the more recent findings of Etgen and Karkanias (1994) that estrogen stimulated oxytocin, which in turn induced the release of NE from the ventromedial hypothalamus.

A second line of evidence linking estrogen to NE activity is the effect of estrogen on adrenergic receptor activity. α_2-receptor activity is altered by fluctuating estrogen levels during the menstrual cycle, after pregnancy, and after menopause. Jones et al. (1983) examined presynaptic α_2 receptors, which inhibit NE release, in human platelets. They found an inverse relationship between α_2-receptor activity and estrogen levels—that is, a cyclic variation in receptor activity that corresponded to the phase of the menstrual cycle. α_2-receptor activity peaked at menses and dropped by almost 80% at midcycle. Presynaptic α_2 receptors inhibit the release of NE. Thus, when estrogen levels were high, there was an increase in NE activity. α_2-receptor activity in male control subjects showed no cyclic variation.

After delivery, the number of platelet α_2 receptors drops significantly, and this drop corresponds to the postpartum decrease in estrogen and progesterone. Platelet α_2 receptors reflect general NE activity. Metz et al. (1983) found that platelet α_2-receptor activity levels in women with "maternity blues" or "postpartum blues" are elevated in comparison with those in control women without depression or women without premenstrual mood changes. This finding suggests that a delay or reduction in the decrease of α_2 activity is associated with the development of maternity blues, which in turn appears to be directly related to the drop in estrogen and progesterone levels that occurs in the immediate postpartum period. Women with depression have also been found to have lower levels of circulating NE on days when they were depressed, compared with days when they were not sad or "blue" (Kuevi et al. 1983).

The drop in estrogen after menopause may also be associated with alterations in noradrenergic function. Best et al. (1992) examined the effect of clonidine, an α-receptor agonist, on variables including 3-methoxy-4-hydroxyphenylethyleneglycol (MHPG [the main metabolite of NE]) levels and α_2 platelet binding in menopausal women before and after receiving a 100-mg implant of estradiol. The estradiol lowered the levels of MHPG but did not alter clonidine α_2 binding.

MHPG levels vary as a function of both age and gender. Halbreich and Lumley (1993) found that women with "endogenous" depressions tended to have MHPG values that were above or below the normal range, whereas men's tended to be within the average range. As women age and estrogen levels drop in postmenopause, MHPG levels and the activity of the NE system also appear to attenuate.

As with other monoamines, the effects of estrogen on NE appear complex. In general, estrogen appears to enhance many aspects of central NE activity, although estrogen can also inhibit NE. NE is thought to be essential in the pathophysiology of many disorders, including mood and anxiety disorders. Thus, estrogen-mediated NE activity may have some role in aspects of psychiatric disorders associated with the menstrual cycle, the postpartum period, and menopause.

Estrogen Modulation of Monoamine Oxidase

In addition to estrogen's direct effects on 5-HT, DA, and NE, estrogen also modulates the activity of these monoamines through its actions on MAO. MAO is responsible for the intracellular enzymatic degradation of monoamines. There are two primary forms of the enzyme: MAO-A and MAO-B. MAO-A is found primarily in the brain, and its primary substrates are epinephrine, NE, and 5-HT. MAO-B is found in serotonergic neurons of the brain, gut, and liver; its primary substrates are tyramine, phenylethylamine, and benzylamine. DA is metabolized by both isoenzymes.

Estrogen appears to have precise effects on MAO in specific regions of the brain. Chevillard and colleagues (1981) found that estrogen administration increased the level of MAO-B but decreased the activity of MAO-A in the locus coeruleus and cerebellum. The inhibition of MAO would be expected to enhance the activity of the monoamines. Likewise, MAO activity was found to be decreased in the amygdala and basomedial hypothalamus in gonadectomized rats treated with estrogen for 3–7 days (Luine et al. 1975). Estrogen appeared to inhibit MAO activity in the midbrain of oophorectomized rats, an effect that reversed when the estrogen was withdrawn.

There appears to be an inverse correlation between menstrual cycle phase and MAO platelet activity. Platelet MAO levels peak at midcycle in rhesus monkeys and reach a nadir during menstruation. In addition, oophorectomized female monkeys appear to show higher MAO platelet activity than do control animals (Redmond et al. 1975). These studies suggest a direct relationship between ovarian steroids and platelet MAO activity.

In human studies, estrogen appears to inhibit MAO activity.

Estrogen agonists have been reported to directly decrease MAO-A activity in neuroblastoma cells (Ma et al. 1995). Similarly, hormone replacement therapy appears to reduce plasma MAO activity in depressed postmenopausal women (Klaiber et al. 1972). However, at least one study in women taking oral contraceptives did not find any significant change in MAO activity as a result of contraceptive therapy (Feldman and Roche 1976).

Clinical Implications

Monoamine neurotransmitters are centrally implicated in most of the significant psychiatric disorders, including major depression and schizophrenia. Given that estrogen can have profound effects on all of the monoamines, it follows that estrogen may be central to some of the gender differences seen in pharmacological treatment response in these disorders.

A higher rate of antidepressant prescriptions for women is consistent with the higher rate of depression in females (Reiger et al. 1990). However, even though women are twice as likely as men to suffer from depression, they are four times as likely to be on an antidepressant. Hohmann (1989) found that women were the recipients of 82% of all antidepressants prescribed, whereas men received only 18% of the prescriptions. This finding may represent a bias in prescribing and/or perhaps might reflect the fact that depressed women are more likely to seek help than are depressed men.

Despite the fact that women are by far the most likely recipients of antidepressant therapy, gender differences in antidepressant tolerability and efficacy have not been given much attention. Nonetheless, gender differences in response to antidepressant treatment are well documented, and estrogen modulation of monoamines may account for many of these differences.

One of the earliest gender differences noted in antidepressant treatment response was that men were more likely than women to respond to antidepressants (Raskin 1974). In 1974, this was probably an accurate assessment, although it is not necessarily true now. A more current statement is that women seem to do less well with certain classes of antidepressants than others.

Women appear to respond to and to tolerate TCAs less well than do men. In a meta-analysis by Hamilton (1995) of multiple imipramine trials involving more than 1,000 patients between 1957 and 1991, 53% of the studies indicated that men were more likely than women to respond to imipramine, while 19% of the studies favored women. No gender difference in response was found in 28% of the studies. When rate of response was examined, about 62% of men were classified as good responders, whereas only 51% of women received this designation. In contrast, some studies of the efficacy of TCAs for the management of pain have favored women (Blumer and Heilbronn 1984; Edelbroeke et al. 1986).

Estrogen may alter the pharmacokinetics of TCAs and other antidepressants. Women tend to have higher serum levels of ami-triptyline than do men receiving the same doses (Preskorn and Mac 1985). The difference in pharmacokinetics may be related to estrogen's influence on the cytochrome P450 system (Hunt et al. 1992) and could partially explain why women are less likely to tolerate TCAs than are men.

There is some evidence that women respond to monoamine oxidase inhibitors (MAOIs) better than do men. Atypical features (i.e., hypersomnia, hyperphagia) may be more prevalent in de-pressed women than in depressed men (Stewart et al. 1993), and a number of studies have suggested that atypical depressions re-spond more favorably to MAOIs than to TCAs (Quitkin et al. 1991, 1993).

Studies of selective serotonin reuptake inhibitors (SSRIs) in the treatment of depression have suggested that women may tol-erate and respond better to these agents than do men. Steiner and colleagues (1993) reported that women appeared to respond to paroxetine better than did men. In a large study of chronic depres-sion involving more than 600 patients, Schatzberg and colleagues (unpublished) found that women were more likely to respond to sertraline than to imipramine. The opposite was true for men. However, when postmenopausal women were evaluated, their response was more similar to that of men. Thus, estrogen status might account for the treatment response differences between pre- and postmenopausal women.

The ability of estrogen to enhance central 5-HT and NE activity while inhibiting MAO would suggest a role for estrogen in the treatment of depression. Unfortunately, very little controlled data exist with which to test this hypothesis. In the 1930s, estrogen was advocated for the treatment of involutional (i.e., geriatric) depression in women. However, reports of its utility were anecdotal.

There is mixed evidence of estrogen's ability to augment the effects of standard antidepressants. Prange et al. (1972) found that estradiol added to imipramine 150 mg/day could speed response, but only by 3 weeks. Imipramine with placebo was as effective as the combination of imipramine and estradiol. Shapira and colleagues (1985) failed to find a difference in response between women who were treated with imipramine 200 mg/day and placebo and those who were treated with the same dose of imipramine and conjugated estrogen at a dose of 3.75 mg/day. In a more recent study, however, Schneider and colleagues (1997) found that women over 60 years of age were far more likely to benefit from fluoxetine if they were also receiving hormone replacement therapy.

Gender differences in the presentation of schizophrenia are, in many respects, intriguing in light of the integral role of dopaminergic systems in the pathophysiology of this illness. Although both men and women have a large peak in onset of schizophrenia during late adolescence, the peak for women is delayed by several years relative to that for men (Maurer and Häfner 1995). Additionally, a second, smaller peak in onset after age 40–45 years is seen in women but not in men (Lindamer et al. 1997). When followed for an average of 8 years after first psychiatric hospitalization, female schizophrenia patients have been shown to have a more benign course than do male patients (Angermeyer et al. 1990). However, older women with schizophrenia have been found to have more positive symptoms than their male counterparts (Lindamer et al. 1997). Riecher-Rossler and Häfner (1993) hypothesized that these gender differences in schizophrenia onset, presentation, and course may be due to estrogen's protecting women from psychosis, an idea that is in concordance with the basic science data showing the antidopaminergic and neuroleptic-like effects of estrogen. In other words, women may have a lower risk of developing psychosis premenopausally because of circulating estrogen, but may have an increased risk of psychotic symptomatology after menopause, when estrogen levels fall. It should be noted, however, that other explanations—for example, certain sociological factors, such as women's earlier average age of marriage, may confer greater amounts of social support during the risk period for the development of psychosis—have been offered to account for these gender discrepancies (Seeman 1997).

There is also significant evidence demonstrating a relationship between premenstrual and postpartum fluctuations in estrogen levels and changes in the risk of psychosis. Women with schizophrenia have been shown to have less psychopathology when measured levels of estradiol were higher during the menstrual cycle (Riecher-Rossler et al. 1994), and to have more psychosis premenstrually, when estrogen levels were low (Hallonquist et al. 1993). Although higher levels of estrogen during pregnancy may protect women from psychosis (Chang and Renshaw 1986), Kendell et al. (1987) found that in a group of 486 female psychiatric patients tracked over a 12-year period, the risk of psychiatric hospitalization as the result of psychosis was 21.7 times greater in the first month and 12.7 times greater in the first 3 months after childbirth in comparison with the risk of hospitalization antepartum. Interestingly, although the risk of admission for psychosis was higher postpartum for women of all diagnoses, the risk was dramatically higher for women with bipolar disorder than for women with schizophrenia. Women with mood disorders may be particularly at risk for the development of psychosis when estrogen levels—and, concomitantly, its antidopaminergic effects—drop precipitously after childbirth. Wieck and colleagues (1991) examined growth hormone secretion in response to apomorphine as a measure of receptor function. They found that DA receptor sensitivity in female affective disorder patients was significantly greater than that in a control group of postpartum women without a psychiatric diagnosis. In fact, two dramatic cases of postpartum psychosis with dyskinesias, one in a woman with schizoaffective disorder and the other in a woman with bipolar disorder, have been attributed to the sudden drop in estrogen levels after childbirth (Vinogradov and Csernansky 1990).

Estrogen's antidopaminergic effects not only may affect the course of schizophrenia and other psychotic disorders but may also have a clinically significant impact on treatment response in these disorders. In a study by Gattaz et al. (1994), women with schizophrenia needed lower doses of neuroleptic medications when their estrogen levels were higher, a finding that points to an additive antipsychotic effect of estrogens. In addition, schizophrenic women generally appear to need lower doses of neuroleptics than do schizophrenic men (Seeman 1995), although this difference in dosage required may result in part from estrogen's inhibition of the cytochrome P450 enzymes responsible for the metabolism of antipsychotics.

Although estrogens may protect against psychosis, they may correspondingly potentiate the risk of neuroleptic-induced extrapyramidal side effects. Compared with men, women have been shown to be more likely to develop parkinsonism and akathisia in response to antipsychotics (Keepers et al. 1983). Furthermore, neuroleptic-related tardive dyskinesia—a condition thought to be associated with supersensitivity of DA receptors—tends to emerge after menopause in women treated with antipsychotics (Kane and Smith 1982) and may be mitigated in men by acute estrogen treatment (Villeneuve et al. 1980).

Finally, several investigators have tested estrogen's utility as an adjunct to antipsychotics for female psychiatric patients. Kulkarni et al. (1996) administered 0.02 mg estradiol and standard antipsychotics to 11 premenopausal female schizophrenia patients and found a greater initial decrease in positive symptoms in these patients compared with subjects treated with standard antipsychotics alone, although the two groups did not differ significantly after a period of 2 months. Lindamer et al. (1997) reported the case of a 49-year-old postmenopausal woman with schizophrenia who was treated with 0.05 mg transdermal estrogen in addition to perphenazine for 5 months. During the time of estrogen treatment, she experienced a decrease in positive symptoms, which rose back to baseline after the estrogen was discontinued. Sichel et al. (1995) prophylactically treated 11 women with histories of severe postpartum mood disorders (7 with psychosis) with high-dose oral estrogen immediately following delivery, tapering the treatment over 4 weeks. They found that 10 of the 11 women remained symptom free both during the study period and during a 1-year follow-up period.

Conclusion

Estrogen appears to be a significant mediator of the gender differences seen in pharmacotherapeutic response of psychiatric disorders such as major depression and schizophrenia. These gender differences are consistent with the complex influence of estrogen on monoamine neurotransmission. Estrogen's effects on monoamines appear to be dose and region specific, sometimes enhancing the activity of a monoamine in one region while inhibiting its activity in another part of the brain. Among the more clinically relevant aspects of estrogen's modulation of monoamines is its ability, under specific conditions, to enhance the activity of 5-HT and NE while inhibiting the activity of MAO and DA. Estrogen appears to influence both the pharmacokinetics and the pharmacodynamics of antidepressant and antipsychotic agents. In addition, given its effects on monoamines, estrogen may have its own intrinsic antidepressant and antipsychotic properties.

The clinical implications of estrogen's apparent antidepressant and antipsychotic properties are unclear. Depressive or psychotic symptoms that are temporally associated with changes in estrogen status, including those symptoms seen in premenstrual, postpartum, and postmenopause syndromes, may eventually become targets for estrogen augmentation of standard therapies. However, at this time, there are not enough data to support the routine use of estrogen supplements in psychiatric disorders, especially given the long-term risks of administering unopposed estrogen, which include malignancy and thrombophlebitis (Lobo 1995). Nonetheless, the exact role of estrogen in the pathophysiology and treatment of major psychiatric syndromes awaits further study.

References

Angermeyer MC, Kuhn L, Goldstein JM: Gender and the course of schizophrenia: differences in treated outcomes. Schizophr Bull 16: 293–307, 1990

Becker JB: Estrogen rapidly potentiates amphetamine-induced striatal dopamine release and rotational behavior during microdialysis. Neurosci Lett 118:169–171, 1990

Bedard P, Dankova J, Boucher R, et al: Effect of estrogens on apomorphine-induced circling behavior in the rat. Can J Physiol Pharmacol 56:538–541, 1978

Bedard PJ, Boucher R, Daigle M, et al: Physiological doses of estradiol can increase lingual dyskinesia and cerebrospinal fluid homovanillic acid in monkeys. Neurosci Lett 58:327–331, 1985

Best NR, Rees MP, Barlow DH, et al: Effect of estradiol implant on noradrenergic function and mood in menopausal subjects. Psychoneuroendocrinology 17:87–93, 1992

Biegon A, McEwen BS: Modulation by estradiol of serotonin receptors in brain. J Neurosci 2:199–205, 1982

Blum M, McEwen BS, Roberts JL: Transcriptional analysis of tyrosine hydroxylase gene expression in the tuberoinfundibular dopaminergic neurons of the rat arcuate nucleus after estrogen treatment. J Biol Chem 262:817–821, 1987

Blumer D, Heilbronn M: Antidepressant treatment for chronic pain: treatment outcome of 1,000 patients with the pain-prone disorder. Psychiatric Annals 14:796–800, 1984

Chang SS, Renshaw DC: Psychosis and Pregnancy. Compr Ther 12:36–41, 1986

Chevillard C, Barden N, Saavedra JM: Estradiol treatment decreases type A and increases type B monoamine oxidase in specific brain stem areas and cerebellum of ovariectomized rats. Brain Res 222: 177–181, 1981

Clarke WP, Goldfarb J: Estrogen enhances a 5-HT$_{1A}$ response in hippocampal slices from female rats. Eur J Pharmacol 160:195–197, 1989

Cone RI, Davis GA, Goy RW: The effects of ovarian steroids on serotonin metabolism within grossly dissected and micro-dissected brain regions in ovariectomized rat. Brain Res Bull 7:639–644, 1981

Di Paolo T, Rouillard C, Bedard P: 17β-Estradiol at a physiological dose acutely increases dopamine turnover in rat brain. Eur J Pharmacol 117:197–203, 1985

Dupont A, Di Paolo T, Gangue B, et al: Effects of chronic estrogen treatment on dopamine concentrations and turnover in discrete brain nuclei of ovariectomized rats. Neurosci Lett 11:69–74, 1981

Edelbroeke PM, Linnsen CG, Zitman FG, et al: Analgesic and antidepressive effects of low-dose amitriptyline in relation to its metabolism in patients with chronic pain. Clin Pharmacol Ther 39:156–162, 1986

Endersby CA, Wilson CA: The effect of ovarian steroids on the accumulation of HJ-labelled monoamines by hypothalamic tissue in vitro. Brain Res 73:3321–3331, 1974

Etgen AM, Karkanias GB: Estrogen regulation of noradrenergic signaling in the hypothalamus. Psychoneuroendocrinology 19:603–10, 1994

Feldman JM, Roche J: Effect of oral contraceptives on platelet monoamine oxidase, monoamine excretion, and adrenocortical function. Clin Pharmacol Ther 20:670–675, 1976

Fink G, Sumner BE, Rosie R, et al: Estrogen control of central neurotransmission: effect on mood, mental state, and memory. Cell Mol Neurobiol 16:325–344, 1996

Gattaz WF, Vogel P, Riecher-Rossler A, et al: Influence of the menstrual cycle phase on the therapeutic response in schizophrenia. Biol Psychiatry 36:137–139, 1994

Gordon JH, Perry KO: Pre- and postsynaptic neurochemical alterations following estrogen-induced striatal dopamine hypo- and hypersensitivity. Brain Res Bull 10:425–428, 1983

Guivarc'h D, Vernier P, Vincent J-D: Sex steroid hormones change the differential distribution of the isoforms of the D_2 dopamine receptor messenger RNA in the rat brain. Neuroscience 69:159–166, 1995

Häfner H, Maurer K, Löffler W, et al: The influence of age and sex on the onset of early course of schizophrenia. Br J Psychiatry 162:80–86, 1993

Halbreich U, Lumley LA: The multiple interactional biological processes that might lead to depression and gender differences in its appearance. J Affect Disord 29:159–173, 1993

Halbreich U, Rojansky N, Palter S, et al: Estrogen augments serotonergic activity in postmenopausal women. Biol Psychiatry 37:434–441, 1995

Hallonquist JD, Seeman MV, Lang M, et al: Variation in symptom severity over the menstrual cycle of schizophrenics. Biol Psychiatry 33:207–209, 1993

Hamilton JA: Sex and gender as critical variables in psychotropic drug research, in Racism and Sexism and Mental Health. Edited by Brown B, Riecker P, Willie C. Pittsburgh, PA, University of Pittsburgh Press, 1995, pp 297–350

Harrer S, Schmidt WJ: Oestrogen modulates dopamine controlled behaviours in the male ferret. Eur J Pharmacol 128:129–132, 1986

Hohmann AA: Gender bias in psychotropic drug prescribing in primary care. Med Care 27:478–490, 1989

Hruska RE, Silbergeld EK: Increased dopamine receptor sensitivity after estrogen treatment using the rat rotational model. Science 208:1446–1468, 1980

Hunt CM, Westerkam WR, Stave GM: Effect of age and gender on the activity of human hepatic CYP3A. Biochem Pharmacol 44:275–283, 1992

Janowsky DS, Fann WE, Davis JM: Monoamines and ovarian hormone–linked sexual and emotional changes. Arch Sex Behav 1:205–218, 1971

Jones SB, Bylund DB, Rieser CA, et al: Alpha2-adrenergic receptor binding in human platelets: alterations during the menstrual cycle. Clin Pharmacol Ther 34:90–96, 1983

Kane JM, Smith JM: Tardive dyskinesia: prevalence and risk factors, 1959–1979. Arch Gen Psychiatry 39:473–481, 1982

Kapur S, Remington G: Serotonin-dopamine interaction and its relevance to schizophrenia. Am J Psychiatry 153:466–476, 1996

Keepers GA, Clappison VJ, Casey DE: Initial anticholinergic prophylaxis for neuroleptic-induced extrapyramidal syndromes. Arch Gen Psychiatry 40:1113–1117, 1983

Kendell RE, Chalmers JC, Platz C: Epidemiology of puerperal psychoses. Br J Psychiatry 150:662–673, 1987

Klaiber EL, Broverman DM, Vogel W, et al: Effects of estrogen therapy on plasma MAO activity and EEG driving responses of depressed women. Am J Psychiatry 128:1492–1498, 1972

Kuevi V, Causon R, Dixson AF, et al: Plasma amine and hormone changes in post-partum blues. Clin Endocrinol (Oxf) 19:39–46, 1983

Kulkarni J, de Castella A, Smith D, et al: A clinical trial of the effects of estrogen in acutely psychotic women. Schizophr Res 20:247–252, 1996

Lindamer LA, Lohr JB, Harris MJ, et al: Gender, estrogen, and schizophrenia. Psychopharmacol Bull 33:221–228, 1997

Lobo RA: Benefits and risks of estrogen replacement therapy. Am J Obstet Gynecol 173 (3 pt 2):882–889, 1995

Luine VN, Khylchevskaya RJ, McEwen BS: Effect of gonadal steroids on activities of monoamine oxidase and choline acetylase in rat brain. Brain Res 86:293–306, 1975

Ma ZQ, Violani E, Villa F, et al: Estrogenic control of monoamine oxidase A activity in human neuroblastoma cells expressing physiological concentrations of estrogen receptor. Eur J Pharmacol 284:171–176, 1995

Maurer K, Häfner H: Methodological aspects of onset assessment in schizophrenia. Schizophr Res 15:265–276, 1995

Mermelstein PG, Becker JB, Surmeier DJ: Estrogen reduces calcium currents in rat nigrostriatal neurons via a membrane receptor. J Neurosci 16:595–604, 1996

Metz A, Stump K, Cowen PJ, et al: Changes in platelet alpha$_2$-adrenoceptor binding post-partum: possible relation to maternity blues. Lancet 1(8323):495–498, 1983

Morissette M, Di Paolo T: Effects of chronic estradiol and progesterone treatments of ovariectomized rats on brain dopamine uptake sites. J Neurochem 60:1876–1883, 1993

Nausieda PA, Koller WC, Weiner WJ, et al: Modification of post-synaptic dopaminergic sensitivity by female sex hormones. Life Sci 25:521–526, 1979

Palermo-Neto J, Dorce VAC: Influences of estrogen and/or progesterone on some dopamine related behavior in rats. Gen Pharmacol 21:83–87, 1990

Paul SM, Axelrod J, Saavedra JM, et al: Estrogen-induced efflux of endogenous catecholamines from the hypothalamus in vitro. Brain Res 178:499–505, 1979

Prange AJ, Wilson IC, Rabon AM, et al: Clinical and theoretical implications of the enhancement of imipramine by tri-iodothyronine in the full spectrum of depressive illnesses, in Recent Advances in the Psychobiology of Depressive Illness. Edited by Williams T, Katz M, Shield JA. Washington, DC, U.S. Government Printing Office, 1972, pp 249–255

Preskorn SH, Mac DS: Plasma levels of amitriptyline: effects of age and sex. J Clin Psychopharmacol 46:276–277, 1985

Quitkin FM, Harrison W, Stewart JW, et al: Response to phenelzine and imipramine in placebo nonresponders with atypical depression: a new application of the crossover design. Arch Gen Psychiatry 48:319–323, 1991

Quitkin FM, Stewart JW, McGrath PJ, et al: Columbia atypical depression: a subgroup of depressives with better response to MAOI than to tricyclic antidepressants or placebo. Br J Psychiatry Suppl 21:30–34, 1993

Raskin A: Age-sex differences in response to antidepressant drugs. J Nerv Ment Dis 159:120–130, 1974

Redmond DE Jr, Murphy DL, Baltu J, et al: Menstrual cycle and ovarian hormone effects on plasma and platelet monoamine oxidase (MAO) and plasma dopamine-beta-hydroxylase (DBH) activities in the rhesus monkey. Psychosom Med 7:417–428, 1975

Reiger DA, Farmer ME, Rae DS, et al: Comorbidity of mental disorders with alcohol and other drug abuse: results from the Epidemiologic Catchment Area (ECA) Study. JAMA 264:2511–2518, 1990

Riecher-Rossler A, Häfner H: Schizophrenia and oestrogens: is there an association? Eur Arch Psychiatry Clin Neurosci 242:323–328, 1993

Riecher-Rossler A, Häfner H, Stumbaum M, et al: Can estradiol modulate schizophrenia symptomatology? Schizophr Bull 20:203–214, 1994

Rojansky N, Halbreich U, Zander K, et al: Imipramine receptor binding and serotonin uptake in platelets of women with premenstrual changes. Gynecol Obstet Invest 31:146–152, 1991

Schneider LS, Small GW, Hamilton SH, et al: Estrogen replacement and response to fluoxetine in a multicenter geriatric depression trial (Fluoxetine Collaborative Study Group). Am J Geriatr Psychiatry 5: 97–106, 1997

Seeman MV: Sex differences in predicting neuroleptic response, in The Prediction of Neuroleptic Response. Edited by Gaebel W, Awad AG. Vienna, Springer-Verlag, 1995, pp 51–64

Seeman MV: Psychopathology in women and men: focus on female hormones. Am J Psychiatry 154:1641–1647, 1997

Shapira B, Oppenheim G, Zohar J, et al: Lack of efficacy of estrogen supplementation to imipramine in resistant female depressives. Biol Psychiatry 20:576–579, 1985

Sichel DA, Cohen LS, Robertson LM, et al: Prophylactic estrogen in recurrent postpartum affective disorder. Biol Psychiatry 38:814–818, 1995

Simerly RB, Chang C, Muramatsu M, et al: Distribution of androgen and estrogen receptor mRNA-containing cells in the rat brain: an in situ hybridization study. J Comp Neurol 294:76–95, 1990

Steiner M, Wheadon DE, Kreider MS, et al: Antidepressant response to paroxetine by gender. Paper presented at the 146th Annual Meeting of the American Psychiatric Association, San Francisco, CA, May 1993

Stewart JW, McGrath PJ, Rabkin JG, et al: Atypical depression: a valid clinical entity? Psychiatr Clin North Am 16:479–495, 1993

Stockert M, DeRobertis E: Effect of ovariectomy and estrogen on [H]imipramine binding to different regions of rat brain. Science 230: 323–325, 1985

Tam WY, Chan MY, Lee PH: The menstrual cycle and changes in platelet 5-HT activity. Psychosom Med 47:352–362, 1985

Van Hartesveldt C, Joyce JN: Effects of estrogen on the basal ganglia. Neurosci Biobehav Rev 10:1–14, 1986

Villeneuve A, Cazejust T, Cote M: Estrogen in tardive dyskinesia in male psychiatric patients. Neuropsychobiology 6:145–151, 1980

Vinogradov S, Csernansky JG: Postpartum psychosis with abnormal movements: dopamine supersensitivity unmasked by withdrawal of endogenous estrogens? J Clin Psychiatry 51:365–366, 1990

Wieck A, Kumar R, Hirst AD, et al: Increased sensitivity of dopamine receptors and recurrence of affective psychosis after childbirth. BMJ 303:613–616, 1991

Wirz-Justice A, Hackman E, Lichsteiner M: The effect of oestradiol dipropionate and progesterone on monoamine uptake in rat brain. J Neurochem 22:187–189, 1974

Xiao L, Becker JB: Effects of estrogen agonists on amphetamine-stimulated striatal dopamine release. Synapse 29:379–391, 1998

Afterword

Ellen Leibenluft, M.D.

What does the future hold for the study of gender and psychiatric illness? Here, as in other areas of clinical psychiatric research, we may soon see the breaking down of some of the nosological barriers that we have so recently erected. It is important to remember that our current diagnostic categories are based solely on symptoms rather than on physiological markers. As physiological markers are identified, our diagnostic system is likely to require significant revision; therefore, taking our current nosological divisions too literally may hamper our research progress.

In other words, we are unlikely to ever identify a neural circuit for, say, DSM-IV 296.2. Instead, given what we know about the organization of the cerebral cortex and about the brain mechanisms underlying animal behavior, we are likely to discover a network of interconnecting circuits, with individual circuits mediating anorexia, decreased concentration, sadness (Reiman et al. 1997), and so forth. As we learn more about the neural events that mediate complex human behaviors, we will be able to identify physiological markers for psychiatric symptoms and illnesses. We may then find that patients who would now all be categorized as having "major depressive disorder" instead suffer from several, distinguishable disorders. Or, alternatively, we may learn that psychiatric syndromes are best characterized by a continuous spectrum of symptom severity, with no clear distinction between illness and health.

Indeed, studies of genetic epidemiology have already begun to challenge our current diagnostic system. Data indicate that neither the distinction between depressive and anxiety disorders (Kendler et al. 1995b) nor that between major depression and more minor depressive disorders (Kendler and Gardner 1998) is consistent with the observed patterns of inheritance for these disorders. For example, data from Kendler et al. (1995b) show that the genetic influences on major depressive disorder and generalized anxiety disorder are, to a large extent, shared. In other words, from a genetic perspective, these two illnesses are not distinct. Similarly, data from Kendler and Gardner (1998) show that depressive symptoms in one twin predict the presence of similar symptoms in a co-twin, even if the index twin's symptoms are of insufficient number or duration to meet the diagnostic criteria for major depression. Thus, these data indicate that depressive symptoms occur along a continuum, and that the current diagnostic distinction between major depression and more mild depressive syndromes may be an arbitrary one.

Just as genetic epidemiology is influencing our view of nosology, so, too, are basic genetic studies changing our perspective on gender. For example, new data indicate that a patient's genetic risk for psychiatric illness may depend not just on whether the patient's parent has the illness, but also on whether the affected parent is the patient's father or mother. Genetic studies in a number of illnesses, including bipolar disorder, are indicating the possible presence of a parent-of-origin effect—that is, a differential risk to the offspring of developing the illness depending on the sex of the affected parent. Such parent-of-origin effects, which have been reported in some forms of deafness, diabetes, and cancer, may result from any one of several mechanisms, including X-linkage, genomic imprinting (when DNA from one parent is deactivated during gametogenesis), mitochondrial inheritance (because mitochondrial DNA occurs in much greater abundance in eggs than in sperm), and trinucleotide repeat expansion (because the extent of the expansion depends partly on the gender of the affected parent) (Hall 1990). Some (e.g., McMahon et al. 1994) but not all (Kato et al. 1996) investigators have found an increased risk of maternal (as opposed to paternal) transmission in bipolar disorder. However, inheritance on chromosome 18, the only putative linkage site in bipolar illness that has been replicated, may be evident only in families with paternal transmission (Gershon et al. 1996; Stine et al. 1995). Thus, the interaction between gender and genes is likely to receive more attention in the future.

Similarly, the three-way interaction between gender, genes, and environment is likely to receive considerably more study in the future. Data from a number of sources indicate that an individual's risk for psychiatric illness includes a significant genetic component. However, these same data leave considerable variance unexplained—variance that is likely to be explained by environmental factors. For example, in a sample of monozygotic twins in which one of each pair was diagnosed with unipolar depression, only 54% of the co-twins also had the illness (Bertelsen et al. 1977). Studies are now beginning to elucidate the relative contribution of environmental and genetic factors to the transmission of psychiatric illness and to identify those environmental factors that are particularly germane (Cadoret et al. 1995; Kendler et al. 1994, 1995). However, few of these studies have examined gender differences in gene–environment interactions. For example, as discussed by Young and Korszun in Chapter 2, the hypothalamic-pituitary-adrenal axis of men and women may respond differently to stressful events, and this fact may have relevance to women's increased risk for depression. Indeed, a recent study showed that the upsurge in major depression among adolescent girls may be due to the fact that, compared with boys, girls have both an increased responsivity to stress and a higher genetic risk (Silberg et al. 1999).

Many of the comments here regarding the future challenges and opportunities in understanding the impact of gender on psychiatric illness are also applicable to other areas of clinical research. In closing, however, it is important to note an issue that is more (although not entirely) unique to this area—namely, the complexity of studying phenomena related to physiological cycles such as the menstrual cycle. All of the chapters in this volume have emphasized the influence that gonadal steroids may have on brain and behavior. In premenopausal women (those at highest risk for most of the illnesses discussed here), levels of gonadal steroids are continually in flux. To study the impact of these hormones on mood or other psychiatric symptoms is, in a sense, to pursue a moving target. Thus, to study the effects of these cycling hormones on psychiatric symptoms, it can be helpful to "clamp" the system pharmacologically with agents such as leuprolide acetate, which suppresses the endogenous secretion of gonadal steroids, and to then "add back" estrogen or progesterone (Schmidt et al. 1991).

Estrogen's cyclicity may help to explain why the authors of some of the chapters in this book have argued that women's high estrogen levels (relative to men's) put them at elevated risk for depression, while the authors of other chapters have noted the potentially antidepressant properties of the hormone. How can estrogen be both "depressogenic" and antidepressant? In premenopausal women, estrogen levels are always either rising or falling, so that estrogen augmentation or withdrawal is continuously occurring. In determining whether estrogen acts as an antidepressant or a depression-inducing agent, the important measure (in the brain, as well as peripherally) may be, not absolute estrogen levels per se, but rather the rate and direction of change (Seeman 1997). This hypothesis is consistent with the evidence—reviewed by Yonkers and Bradshaw in Chapter 4—indicating that the perimenopause, a time when hormonal shifts can be particularly dramatic, may be associated with an increase in mood lability.

Finally, estrogen, like other psychotropic agents, is likely to have complex actions, so that it may be antidepressant with regard to some symptoms (e.g., improved concentration) and "depressogenic" with regard to others (e.g., increased reactivity to stress). And, as indicated by a number of authors, it is important to remember that there is a great deal of interindividual variability, among both men and women, in sensitivity to the psychotropic effects of gonadal steroids and, probably, to the effects of other hormones as well. Future study will teach us how to identify sensitive individuals and will help us understand the mechanisms underlying this variability in the population.

As the chapters in this book attest, tremendous progress has been made in our understanding of whether, and how, a patient's gender influences his or her risk for psychiatric illness and the course that the illness might take. The rate of progress in this area has accelerated rapidly within the past decade; this progress has been fueled in large part by the awareness that, for both clinical and scientific reasons, gender differences are an important area of study. Of course, much remains unknown, particularly about gender differences in treatment response and about the mechanisms underlying the clinical differences that we observe. We look forward to continued progress in the future, and to the benefits that that progress will bring to our patients—male and female alike—who suffer from these illnesses.

References

Bertelsen A, Harvald B, Hauge M: A Danish twin study of manic-depressive disorders. Br J Psychiatry 130:330–351, 1977

Cadoret RJ, Yates WR, Troughton E, et al: Genetic-environmental interaction in genesis of aggressivity and conduct disorders. Arch Gen Psychiatry 52:916–924, 1995

Gershon ES, Badner JA, Detera-Wadleigh SD, et al: Maternal inheritance and chromosome 18 allele sharing in unilineal bipolar illness pedigrees. Am J Med Genet 67:202–207, 1996

Hall J: Genomic imprinting: review and relevance to human diseases. Am J Hum Genet 46:857–873, 1990

Kato T, Winokur G, Coryell W, et al: Parent-of-origin effect in transmission of bipolar disorder. Am J Med Genet 67:546–550, 1996

Kendler KS, Gardner CO Jr: Boundaries of major depression: an evaluation of DSM-IV criteria. Am J Psychiatry 155:172–177, 1998

Kendler KS, Walters EE, Truett KR, et al: Sources of individual differences in depressive symptoms: analysis of two samples of twins and their families. Am J Psychiatry 151:1605–1614, 1994

Kendler KS, Walters EE, Neale MC, et al: The structure of the genetic and environmental risk factors for six major psychiatric disorders in women. Arch Gen Psychiatry 52:374–383, 1995

McMahon FJ, Stine OC, Meyers DA, et al: Patterns of maternal transmission in bipolar affective disorder. Am J Hum Genet 56:1277–1286, 1994

Reiman EM, Lane RD, Ahern GL, et al: Neuroanatomical correlates of externally and internally generated human emotion. Am J Psychiatry 154:918–925, 1997

Schmidt PJ, Nieman LK, Grover GN, et al: Lack of effect of induced menses on symptoms in women with premenstrual syndrome. N Engl J Med 324:1174–1179, 1991

Seeman MV: Psychopathology in women and men: focus on female hormones. Am J Psychiatry 154:1641–1647, 1997

Silberg J, Pickles A, Rutter M, et al: The influence of genetic factors and life stress on depression among adolescent girls. Arch Gen Psychiatry 56:225–232, 1999

Stine OC, Xu J, Koskela R, et al: Evidence for linkage of bipolar disorder to chromosome 18 with a parent-of-origin effect. Am J Hum Genet 57:1384–1394, 1995

Index

*Page numbers printed in **boldface** type refer to tables or figures.*

Dosages *(continued)*
  of estradiol with progestin for mood disorders, 116
  of estrogen and dopamine modulation, 141
  of estrogen and mood changes, 121
  of estrogen in oral contraceptives, 93
  of neuroleptics for schizophrenia, 153
  of progestin in oral contraceptives and mood, 126–127
Dysphoria, and oral contraceptives, 125. *See also* Premenstrual dysphoric disorder

Elderly, and hypothalamic-pituitary-adrenal axis, 34. *See also* Aging
Environment
  interaction between gender, genetics, and, 163
  research on sex differences in brain morphology, 2
Estradiol. *See also* Transdermal 17 β-estradiol
  corticosterone stress response and, 40
  menstrual cycle and, 92
  mood disorders and, 108, 109
Estrogen. *See also* Hormone replacement therapy; Oral contraceptives
  administration of exogenous, 92–95
  Alzheimer's disease and, 21
  anxiety and, 63–64, 75, 76, 77
  cerebral blood flow and, 18
  cyclicity of as difficulty in research, 163–164
  dopaminergic system and, 140–145
  dosage of and mood changes, 121
  hypothalamic-pituitary-adrenal axis and, 40–41, 43, 46–47
  monoamine oxidase modulation and, 148–154
  mood disorders and, 97–116, 127–128
  norepinephrine modulation and, 145–148
  prevalence of prescribed use of, 91
  serotonergic system and, 95–97, 137–140
Estrone and estrone sulfate, 92, 110, 111, 116
Estrus cycle, reproductive hormones and anxiety, 66–67
Ethinyl estradiol, 92–93, 108
Exercise, progesterone and stress response, 45

Fawn-Hooded rat strain, 61
Fear, conditioned and unconditioned in animal models, 62
Fetus, sex hormones and brain development, 3–4, 72. *See also* Pregnancy
Fluoxetine, 113, 151
Flutamide, 65
Functional imaging, definition of, 3
Functional lateralization, of brain hemispheres, 16–17

Hispanic-American women, and
effects of estrogen on mood,
108
Homeostasis, and stress, 31–32
Homovanillic acid, 141
Hormone replacement therapy
(HRT). *See also* Estrogen
conjugated estrogens in, 93–94
fluoxetine and, 113
monoamine oxidase activity
and, 149
mood and, 111–112, 127–128
Hospital Adjustment Scale
(HAS), 113
Hypercortisolemia, 34, 37, 39, 44
Hyperthyroidism, 68–69
Hypertriglyceridemia, 93
Hypothalamic-pituitary-adrenal
(HPA) axis. *See also*
Hypothalamus
animal studies of regulation of,
39–42
lactation and, 70
overview of regulation, 33–34
prenatal stress and anxiety, 72
sex differences in depression
and, 34–39
sex differences in regulation
of, 42–48
stress and activation of, 31–32
Hypothalamus, sex hormones
and development of, 4. *See
also* Hypothalamic-pituitary-
adrenal axis
Hypothyroidism, 68, 69
Hysterectomy, and estrogen, 99,
108, 127–128, 140

Imipramine
estrogen and serotonin system,
139

gender and response to, 150,
151
Immune function, and
pregnancy, 68
Infants, and planum temporale
asymmetry, 15. *See also*
Neonates
Interindividual variability, and
gender-related research, 164
Intracranial volume, and height,
13–15

Lactation, and anxiety, 69–70
Learned helplessness, 62
Leuprolide acetate, 45, 163–164
Levonorgestrel, 108, 126

Magnetic resonance imaging
(MRI) studies, of sex
differences
adult brain morphology and, 9
brain development and, 7
development of cellular
structure of brain and, 6
glucose metabolism and, 19
hemispheric lateralization and,
17
intracranial volume and
height, 13–15
Major depressive disorder
(MDD). *See also* Depression
estrogen and, 109–110,
112–114, 115, 127, 128
genetic influences on, 162
Maturation, gender and brain
growth, 6–8
Maudsley Reactive rat strain, 61
Medroxyprogesterone, and mood
disorders, **94,** 95, 111, 116,
120
Megestrol acetate, **94,** 95

Neuropeptide Y, 70
Neurosteroids, 55, 57
Neurotransmitters, and estrogen
    modulation of monoamine,
    148–154
Non-placebo-controlled studies,
    of estrogen and mood
    disorders, 111–112
Norepinephrine
    estrogen and modulation of,
    145–148
    stress and pathophysiology of
    anxiety and depression,
    58
Norethindrone and
    norethindrone acetate, **94,** 95,
    109, 116
Norgestrel, **94,** 95, 125

Obsessive-compulsive disorder,
    65, 68
Oral contraceptives. *See also*
    Estrogen; Progestins
    cortisol response to stress and,
    43
    forms of estrogens used in,
    92–93
    mood disorders and, 121–127
Oxytocin
    anxiety and stress response, 57
    estrogen and anxiolytic effects
    of, 63
    lactation and, 69–70
    obsessive-compulsive disorder
    and, 65

Panic disorder
    estrogen treatment of patients
    with, 64
    lactation and, 69
    pregnancy and, 68

Paraventricular nucleus of
    hypothalamus (PVN), 34
Parent-of-origin effects, in
    genetics, 162
Parkinsonism, and
    antipsychotics, 153
Perimenopause
    definition of, 97
    estrogen and mood disorders,
    100–102, 110–111, 127,
    164
Perphenazine, 153
Placebo-controlled studies
    of estrogen and menopausal
    mood disorders, 99–111,
    115
    of oral contraceptives and
    mood disorders, **122–124**
Planum temporale asymmetry, 15
Positron emission tomography
    (PET) studies, of sex
    differences
    depression and, 23
    glucose metabolism and, 18,
    19
    hemispheric lateralization and,
    17
Postpartum depression, 112, 114,
    147
Postpartum psychosis, 153
Posttraumatic stress disorder
    (PTSD), 47, 72
Pregnancy. *See also* Fetus
    hypothalamic-pituitary-
    adrenal axis and, 44
    neurosteroids and, 55
    obsessive-compulsive disorder
    and, 65
    psychosis and, 152
    reproductive hormones and
    anxiety, 68–69

Premenstrual dysphoric disorder (PMDD)
  estrogen and, 114
  imipramine binding and, 139
  progesterone and, 45
Premenstrual syndrome (PMS)
  estrogen as treatment for, 112
  oral contraceptives and, 126, 128
  progestins as treatment for mood disorders and, 120
Prenatal stress, sex differences in developmental response to, 72
Progesterone. *See also* Progestins
  cortisol and, 43–44
  exercise stress response and, 45
  exogenous administration of, 94–95
  gender and anxiety, 64–65, 77
  hypothalamic-pituitary-adrenal axis and, 41, 46
  norepinephrine and, 147
  serotonergic system and, 95–97
Progestins. *See also* Oral contraceptives; Progesterone
  administration of exogenous, 92–95
  menopausal mood disorders and, 116–121
  prevalence of prescribed use of, 91
Prolactin, 70, 140
Proopiomelanocorticotropin (POMC), 33
Pruning, and development of neocortex, 6, 8
Psychosis, 152, 154

Psychosocial events. *See also* Social factors
  mood symptoms of menopause and, 98
  oral contraceptives and mood, 128
Puberty, and depression in women, 48

Reproductive hormones. *See also* Sex hormones
  animal models for anxiety and, 59–62
  cellular mechanisms of action, 53–57
  gender and effects of on anxiety, 63–70
  sex differences in anxiety-related neurochemical systems, 73–76
Resting state, and sex differences in glucose metabolism, 19
Roman Low-Avoidance rat strain, 61

Schizoaffective disorder, 153
Schizophrenia
  gender and cerebral volume, 2
  gender differences in presentation of, 151–152
  gender differences in treatment response, 153
  pruning in cerebral cortex, 8
  sex differences in brain morphology and, 21–23
Seizures, 75
Selective serotonin reuptake inhibitors (SSRIs), 150–151
Serotonin reuptake blockers, 59